ANTICIPATE

RESPOND

RECOVER

ANTICIPATE RESPOND RECOVER

Healthcare Leadership and Catastrophic Events

K. Joanne McGlown • Phillip D. Robinson • Editors

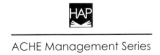

ACHE Management Series

Reprinted October 2020

Library of Congress Cataloging-in-Publication Data

Anticipate, respond, recover : healthcare leadership and catastrophic events / edited by K. Joanne McGlown and Phillip Robinson.
   p. ; cm.
 Includes bibliographical references and index.
 ISBN 978-1-56793-366-6 (alk. paper)
 1. Emergency medical services--United States. 2. Hospitals--Administration. I. McGlown, K. Joanne, editor. II. Robinson, Phillip, editor.
 [DNLM: 1. Disaster Planning--organization & administration--United States. 2. Hospitals--United States. 3. Hospital Administration--methods--United States. 4. Organizational Policy--United States. WX 186]
 RA645.5.A546 2011
 362.18--dc22
                  2010051669

The paper used in this publication meets the minimum requirements of American National Standard for Information Sciences—Permanence of Paper for Printed Library Materials, ANSI Z39.48-1984. ∞ ™

Acquisitions editor: Eileen Lynch; Project manager: Eduard Avis; Cover designer: Scott Miller; Layout: Scott Miller

Found an error or a typo? We want to know! Please e-mail it to hap1@ache.org, and put "Book Error" in the subject line.

For photocopying and copyright information, please contact Copyright Clearance Center at www.copyright.com or at (978) 750–8400.

Health Administration Press
A division of the Foundation of the American College of
   Healthcare Executives
300 S. Riverside Plaza, Suite 1900
Chicago, IL 60606-6698
(312) 424–2800

This book is dedicated to all of the committed emergency responders and healthcare workers who are integral to the preparation for and response to crisis situations. Their selfless commitment to our safety and security often goes unnoticed until we are in the midst of a challenging situation. Leaders in planning and responding to manmade and natural disasters are similarly overlooked. We often forget that these responders and healthcare providers are often also victims of the same event, and that the impact on them can be long lasting and traumatic. They deserve not only our ongoing thanks, but also our support and understanding of their special role in our society.

The authors would like to specifically dedicate this book to those who were part of the response and recovery efforts in Hurricanes Katrina and Ike, and to those whose lives were forever changed by the impact of these storms.

Partial proceeds from this book will be donated to the School of Rural Public Health at the Texas A&M Health Science Center to assist them in the development of the future leaders and public health professionals who will be integral to our response to the critical challenges yet to come.

Far and away the best prize that life offers is the chance to work hard at work worth doing.

Theodore Roosevelt, Labor Day speech, September 7, 1903, Syracuse, NY

And I heard the Lord saying, Whom shall I send? Who will go for me? And I answered Here Am I. Send Me.

Isaiah 6:8

Contents

Disasters in Arkansas: The Hospital's and Hospital Association's Viewpoint—An Interview with Angela L. Richmond, Kirk Reamey, and Beth Ingram 173

Preface

As we go to press with this book, media coverage of scientific knowledge gained over the past few years has increased our awareness of Earth changes. On December 20, 2010, the Associated Press wrote "2010's World Gone Wild: Quakes, Floods, Blizzards," calling 2010 "the deadliest year in more than a generation. More people were killed worldwide by natural disasters this year than have been killed in terrorism attacks in the past 40 years combined." Through November 30, 2010 nearly 260,000 people died of natural disasters in 2010, compared to 15,000 in 2009, according to Geneva-based insurance giant Swiss Re (Bell and Borenstein 2010).

Andreas Schraft, vice president of catastrophic perils for Swiss Re, stated that "disasters from the Earth are pretty much constant," and Craig Fugate, the director of the U.S. Federal Emergency Management Agency (FEMA) stated "It just seemed like it was back-to-back, and it came in waves." Even the extremes "are changed in an extreme fashion," said Greg Holland, director of the earth system laboratory at the National Center for Atmospheric Research. FEMA declared a record number of major disasters for 2010, 79 as of December 14th. The average year has 34 (Bell and Borenstein 2010).

Scientists and disaster experts agree that "the hand of man made this a particularly deadly, costly, extreme and weird year for everything from wild weather to earthquakes. The excessive amount of extreme weather that dominated 2010 is a classic sign of man-made global warming that climate scientists have long warned about" (Bell and Borenstein 2010). It was also a year of man-made technological catastrophes; all while the world's population is moving to riskier megacities on fault zones and flood prone areas.

Every disaster and catastrophic event has a medical impact. Large-scale events can affect entire populations and require a coordinated response among public health services.

It is the responsibility of healthcare executives to know as much about disaster preparedness, response, recovery, and mitigation as they know about healthcare finance, insurance, and medical staff credentialing. To trivialize or overlook this one component of education and knowledge can, in the blink of an eye, incapacitate a healthcare facility or delivery system, placing all in it in great jeopardy and danger. Let this be the year that you, the healthcare leader, become as prepared and aware as the CEOs and healthcare leaders who boldly participated in sharing their stories and enriching this book with their truth and insight.

HOW THIS BOOK IS ORGANIZED

This book is designed to be a quick read of the most important information a healthcare leader needs to prepare for, respond to, recover from, and mitigate disasters and large-scale catastrophic events. It is written in a simplistic fashion, to allow you to open the book to any section and garner nuggets of wisdom.

The book is divided into four primary parts:

I. Introduction and Preparedness (Chapters 1-3)
II. Response (Chapters 4)
III. Recovery (Chapters 5-8)
IV. Lessons Learned, Cases, and Real Life Experiences (Chapter 9)

Mitigation is a primary topic of this book, and is reflected throughout the chapters. A number of sidebars and exhibits in each chapter provide more detailed information on the topics covered.

PART 1

This section describes disasters and catastrophes and introduces the healthcare leader to the organization of our nation for response to such events. Whether local, state, or federal level involvement is required, the processes for preparedness, response, and recovery are based on the National Response Framework. These chapters also describe preparedness planning, both internally and externally.

Chapter 1 Disasters and Catastrophes Defined. Statistics illustrate that disasters are increasing in frequency and severity, concurrently increasing the risk to healthcare organizations. The conundrum of terminology is discussed and the impact of catastrophic events on healthcare and related business entities is introduced.

Chapter 2 Organizing for Disasters. It is important to understand the state and federal direction and roles in catastrophe planning. This chapter describes the roles of and relationships among the various federal guidance programs, such as the National Incident Managment System and the National Strategy for Homeland Security. The agencies that support this response, from the local to the federal level, are discussed.

Chapter 3 Preparedness Planning for Catastrophic Health Events. Awareness of business crisis and continuity management principles is essential when you prepare your facility, internally and externally, for catastrophic events. Strengthening resilience and building coalitions are critical to the sustainability of healthcare services.

PART II

This section discusses the challenges faced by leaders when their organizations must respond to a disaster.

Chapter 4 Responding: You're In This Alone. In this chapter, the authors and others who have led their organizations through catastrophic events share anecdotes about their challenges and offer leadership wisdom. Identifying and grooming disaster leaders and having an awareness of the overwhelming number of internal issues that must be faced during a disaster are critical to leadership preparedness. Don Smithburg has contributed "A Pocket Book Primer for the Executive: Ten Steps in Disaster Planning," which should prove of great value to healthcare leaders preparing for potential catastrophic events.

PART III

This section describes the recovery phase.

Chapter 5 Recovery: The Good, the Bad, and the Ugly. Recovery in the aftermath of a critical event doesn't occur without proper and extensive planning and preparation. This chapter discusses recovery and sustainability, identifies resources, and reviews key internal issues that healthcare organizations need to address.

Chapter 6 Financial Planning for Catastrophic Events

Chapter 7 Financial Actions During and After the Catastrophe

These chapters provide an in-depth review of the importance of solid financial planning for catastrophic events. Building awareness of employee roles, estimating costs, and providing adequate coverage to insure such an event are initial steps. Chapter 7 covers financial actions to activate recovery and protection of the facility and its operations.

Chapter 8 What's In Our Future? This chapter provides an overview of challenges we may be facing in the near future concerning Earth changes—their impact on populations and on the provision of healthcare. The literature is flush with scientific articles and data from credible sources warning of the increasing tempo and destructive potential of disasters and catastrophic events. The challenges facing our profession are vast, and continuity of care among healthcare providers is fully the responsibility of the healthcare CEO and governance leaders. There is time to prepare for future catastrophic events, if we heed the clear warnings and remain knowledgeable of the threats. Changing an organization's culture is one of the most difficult tasks facing healthcare leaders; developing a "disaster culture" within your healthcare organization is the most valuable gift a leader can provide. The time to begin is long overdue.

PART IV

The final part of this book consists of lessons learned from those who managed their organizations through a variety of disasters. Their "real world" experiences provide exceptional advice to current and future healthcare leaders. From CEOs and other healthcare leaders of large urban medical centers to university-based systems to not-for-profit and for-profit environments, these leaders share their timely messages and wisdom to encourage preparedness at all stages.

Part I

INTRODUCTION AND PREPAREDNESS

 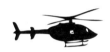

CHAPTER 1

Disasters and Catastrophes Defined

The United States is a volatile land, with risks at every turn. We face the following risks:

- Floods occur in all 50 states and all U.S. territories (FEMA 2010c).
- Earthquakes have occurred in 43 U.S. states in the past 30 years (USGS 2009a).
- On average, five hurricanes strike the United States every three years (AOML 2010).
- Wildfires occur annually (USGS 2010).
- Tornados affect every state (every state has had at least one tornado) (Climate Services Monitoring Division 2010).
- The United States is home to 65 active or potentially active volcanoes (National Academies Press 2000).
- Landslides occur in every state (USGS 2009b).
- Almost 14,000 oil spills are reported each year in the United States (NSTC 2003).
- Each year, fire kills more Americans than all other natural disasters combined (NESEC n.d.).

Concerning earthquakes specifically,

- 39 states in the last 100 years experienced damage from earthquakes (HP and SCORE 2007),
- 90 percent of Americans live in seismically active areas (IINC 2006), and
- only 25 percent of homeowners in California have earthquake insurance (Insure.com 2009).

EMERGENCIES, DISASTERS, CATASTROPHES, AND CRISES

With a plethora of different definitions for *disaster*, it is understandable that health-care leaders are unsure of the terminology when it comes to describing an event and often use these terms interchangeably.

One definition of *disaster* stated that it was "a calamitous event, especially one occurring suddenly and causing great loss of life, damage or hardship" (American Heritage Dictionary 2006). A synonym was "catastrophe." How can a disaster be a catastrophe? Are they one and the same? The business and insurance industries define a catastrophic event differently than an emergency manager does. In fact, the *catastrophe* definition in the business and insurance industries has changed over time. Exhibit 1.1 provides published definitions, but it may be easier to focus on the way academia clarifies these terms.

Exhibit 1.1: The Conundrum of Definitions

Definitions (*American Heritage Dictionary* 2006) are confusing and not much help in the delineation or categorization of an event. The two definitions that follow illustrate this conundrum clearly:

- Disaster: an occurrence causing widespread destruction and distress; a catastrophe
- Emergency: a serious situation or occurrence that happens unexpectedly and demands immediate action

e· mer·gen·cy: *noun*
  1. A sudden urgent, usually unexpected occurrence or occasion requiring immediate action
  2. A state, esp. of need for help or relief, created by some unexpected event: a weather emergency, a financial emergency

---

Synonyms:

Extremity, plight. EMERGENCY, CRISIS, STRAITS refer to dangerous situations. An EMERGENCY is a situation demanding immediate action. A CRISIS is a vital or decisive turning point in a condition or state of affairs, and everything depends on the outcome of it. STRAIT suggests a pressing situation, often one of need or want.

Source: Dictionary.com Unabridged. Based on the *Random House Dictionary*, Random House, Inc., 2010, s.v. "Emergency."

e· mer·gen·cy

1. A serious situation or occurrence that happens unexpectedly and demands immediate attention
2. A condition of urgent need for action or assistance; a state of emergency

Source: *The American Heritage Dictionary of the English Language*, 4th ed., s.v. "Emergency."

e· mer·gen·cy

1. An unforeseen combination of circumstances or the resulting state that calls for immediate action
2. An urgent need for assistance or relief

Source: *Merriam-Webster's Dictionary of Law*, 1996, Merriam-Webster, Inc., s.v. "Emergency."

e· mer·gen·cy: An unforeseen combination of circumstances or the resulting state that calls for immediate action

Source: *Merriam-Webster's Medical Dictionary*, 2002. Merriam-Webster, Inc., s.v. "Emergency."

dis·as·ter: *noun*

1. A calamitous event, especially one occurring suddenly and causing great loss of life, damage, or hardship, as a flood, airplane crash, or business failure

Synonyms:

DISASTER, CALAMITY, CATASTROPHE, CATACLYSM refer to adverse happenings often occurring suddenly and unexpectedly. A DISASTER may be caused by carelessness, negligence, bad judgment, or the like, or by natural forces as a hurricane or flood. CALAMITY suggests great affliction, either personal or general; the emphasis is on the grief or sorrow caused. CATASTROPHE refers esp. to the tragic outcome of a personal or public situation; the emphasis is on the destruction or irreplaceable loss: the catastrophe of a defeat in battle. CATACLYSM, physically an earth-shaking change, refers to a personal or public upheaval of unparalleled violence.

Source: Dictionary.com Unabridged. Based on the *Random House Dictionary*, Random House, Inc., 2010, s.v. "Disaster."

(continued)

---

dis·as·ter (from the French "désastre"; the Italian "disastro")

1. An occurrence causing widespread destruction and distress; a catastrophe
2. A grave misfortune

Source: The *American Heritage Dictionary of the English Language*, 4th ed., s.v. "Disaster."

dis·as·ter

1580, from M.Fr. désastre (1564), from It. disastro "ill-starred," from dis- "away, without" + astro "star, planet," from L. astrum, from Gk. astron. The sense is astrological, of a calamity blamed on an unfavorable position of a planet.

Source: Online Etymology Dictionary, s.v. "Disaster."

ca·tas·tro·phe: *noun*

1. A sudden and widespread disaster; any misfortune, mishap or failure

Source: Dictionary.com Unabridged. Based on the *Random House Dictionary*, Random House, Inc., 2010 s.v. "Catastrophe."

ca·tas·tro·phe

- A great, often sudden calamity
- A sudden violent change in the earth's surface, a cataclysm
- From the Greek *catastrophe, an overturning, ruin, conclusion*

Source: The *American Heritage Dictionary of the English Language*, 4th ed., 2006. Houghton Mifflin Harcourt, s.v. "Catastrophe."

ca·tas·tro·phe

From 1540, "reversal of what is expected" from Gk. katastrephein "to overturn," from kata "down" + strephein "turn." Extension to "sudden disaster" is first recorded in 1748. Catastrophism as a geological or biological theory is from 1869.

Source: Online Etymology Dictionary, s.v. "Catastrophe."

ca·tas·tro·phe

- Death (as from an inexplicable cause) before, during, or after an operation

Source: Merriam-Webster's Medical Dictionary, s.v. "Catastrophe."

Considering a number of variables makes it much easier to see the differences in these terms, guiding us to use them more appropriately. For the purpose of this book, the terms *emergency, disaster,* and *catastrophe* are defined as Exhibit 1.2 shows.

An emergency is a common event. An example of an emergency might be an accident resulting in a broken bone, heart attack, or stroke. Although the event

Exhibit 1.2 How Bad Is It?

	Routineness/ Severity	Impact/ Resources	Social Order/ Psyche
Emergency	Routine, adverse events	None outside the affected individual or family	No disruption or long-term effect
Disaster	Nonroutine, severe	Community-wide impact; may require resource assistance	Disruption to social order or psyche of area or region
Catastrophe	Unusually extreme, rare events	Effect on entire nation and/or parts of the world; requires extensive resource assistance	Long-term disruption to the social order, security, or psyche of a nation or its people

may have a severe effect on the patient or immediate family members, it is routinely handled well by the local emergency medical services system. An emergency causes no disruption to the social order or psyche of the community or population.

A disaster is a severe event such as a massive flood, destructive tornado or hurricane, or human-caused or terrorist attack. The community may be affected, and resource need may overwhelm the local area, requiring outside assistance from the state or even federal government (as occurs with a presidential disaster declaration). These events disrupt the social order, psyche, and sense of security of those living in the region, and memories of such events may persist for generations.

A catastrophe is an unusually extreme, rare event that affects an entire nation or part of the world. Recent catastrophic events have included the events of September 11, 2001 in the United States, the Banda Aceh earthquake and resulting tsunami, the recent massive earthquakes in Haiti and Chile, and extensive, severe flooding in Pakistan and other areas of the world. These events require extensive resource assistance from outside the region and a global response. The damage to the social order, psyche, and security of the country or countries affected may be profound and prolonged.

Based on the United Nations definition, natural catastrophes are classified as *great* if a region's ability to help itself is distinctly overtaxed, making supraregional or international assistance necessary. As a rule, this is the case when there are thousands of fatalities, hundreds of thousands are left homeless, and/or overall losses are of exceptional proportions given the economic circumstances of the country concerned. In terms of our great natural catastrophe statistics, this means specifically:

- ◆ Number of fatalities exceeds 2,000 and/or
- ◆ number of homeless exceeds 200,000 and/or
- ◆ overall losses exceed 5 percent of that country's per capita GDP and/or
- ◆ the country is dependent on international aid.

Since 1950, 285 catastrophes have fulfilled these criteria, with approximately 30 percent meeting all criteria.

A natural catastrophe can only come about if a society is not sufficiently prepared for an extreme natural event. Global changes have meant increased vulnerability nearly everywhere (Wirtz 2010, used with permission).

DISASTERS ARE INCREASING IN FREQUENCY AND SEVERITY

Globally, disasters have increased in frequency and severity. Between 1994 and 2003 (the last decade for which we have statistics), more than 2.5 billion people were affected by natural disasters—a 60 percent increase over the two previous decades. And in the United States alone, where we average about 400 disasters with damage a year, the numbers from 1994 to 2003 were 25 percent higher than the average for the previous decade. Exhibit 1.3 lists the U.S. states with the most federal disaster declarations since 1953 (CRED 2008).

Exhibit 1.3 States with Most Disasters

State	Disaster Declarations
Texas	83
California	74
Florida	61
Oklahoma	61
New York	57
Louisiana	55

Source: FEMA (2010a).

The 2005 Atlantic hurricane season remains the busiest in recorded history. Exhibit 1.4 shows the records that were surpassed that year.

Publications overflow with statistics of the negative effects of disasters worldwide.

- The death toll from disasters over the last 50 years exceeds 12 million persons, with billions affected. Economic costs are estimated as high as $4 trillion (Sundnes and Birnbaum 2003).
- On average, one disaster per week requires international assistance (Veenema 2003).
- During the past 20 years, natural disasters have killed at least 3 million people and have affected 800 million more (Bruntland 2003).
- The Spanish Flu outbreak of 1918–19 was the worst pandemic in modern times. An estimated 17 million people died in India—about 5 percent of India's population at the time. Almost 22 percent of troops in the Indian Army died, and it is estimated that between 2 and 5 percent of the global population at the time died.

The Federal Emergency Management Agency (FEMA) has recorded 1,826 disasters since 1953, an average of 32 federally declared disasters per year (FEMA 2010a). Yet, the United States has suffered few civilian disasters on a massive scale. Fewer than ten civilian disasters in the United States have had fatality rates exceeding 1,000, and "only about 10–15 disasters per year have resulted in more than 40 injuries" (Wright 1976).

Exhibit 1.4 Records: Hurricanes and Tropical Storms

Record Title	Previous Record	2005 Record	New Record
Most named tropical storms	21 (1993)	28	Unchanged
Number of hurricanes	12 (1969)	15	Unchanged
Major hurricanes hitting the United States	3 (2004)	4	Unchanged (3 in 2008)
Category 5 intensity (> 155 mph)	2 (1960 and 1961)	4	Unchanged
Costliest	$26.5 billion (1992 dollars), Hurricane Andrew	$80 billion (2005 dollars), Hurricane Katrina	

Source: Data from NOAA (2006; 2010).

However, most U.S. disasters are not of extraordinary magnitude, and many of the logistics problems faced in disasters are caused not by shortages of medical resources, but by failures to coordinate their distribution. The United States possesses an abundance of resources. Except in poor, rural areas, the United States experienced supply shortages in only 6 percent of hospitals involved in disasters and personnel shortages in 2 percent of them (Wright 1976).

The expanding U.S. population "has migrated to hazard-prone areas, and the way America builds too often invites disasters," and "we're building our communities in ways that aren't compatible with the natural perils we have" (Miletti 1999).

Yet, Glantz and Qian Ye (2010) state that "most people don't choose to live in hazardous places at high risk of climate, water, or weather extremes; usually, they do not have the financial means to avoid such conditions" (37) and that "at risk areas will likely increase in number as warming of the global atmosphere continues to go relatively unchecked" (45).

In the United States, our vulnerability is increasing.

◆ Domestically, "25–50 million people live in floodplains that have been developed as living and working environments; and by 2010, 60 percent of the U.S. population may be living within 50 miles of either the East or West coasts" (Landeman 2005).

◆ Thirty-nine U.S. states are seismically active, and at least 70 million people face significant risk of death or injury from earthquakes (Landeman 2005). In fact, from 1974 to 2003, 42 states had at least one earthquake with a magnitude of 3.5 or greater (USGS 2009).

The following socioeconomic factors can turn natural events into devastating catastrophes (Wirtz 2010, 35):

◆ Population growth
  • Our current population is 6.8 billion. According to UN forecasts, the population will climb to more than 9 billion by 2050.
◆ Settlement and industrialization of highly exposed regions
  • One-third of the world's population live within 50 kilometers of the nearest coast.
◆ Concentration of population and values
  • The number of cities worldwide with more than 1 million inhabitants has risen from around 80 in 1950 to about 400 today, and more than 50 percent of the world's population lives in cities. By 2030, it will be over 60 percent.
◆ Vulnerability of modern societies

◆ Rising insurance density and global networking
  • Climate change has led to a rise in extreme weather events.

BUSINESS LOSS: A WAKE-UP CALL FOR HEALTHCARE

The insured share of total economic losses from weather-related catastrophes has increased from a negligible fraction in the 1950s to 24 percent in the last decade. The ratio has climbed more quickly in the United States, where more than 40 percent of the total disaster losses in the 1990s were insured. Disasters affecting healthcare and clinical practice come in all forms, and any disaster poses a risk to a community's healthcare services.

Exhibit 1.5 illustrates the percentage of U.S. organizations that have experienced a significant business interruption as a result of a natural or man-made disaster; it also shows that man-made disasters are far more common than natural disasters. Exhibit 1.6 shows the global toll of natural disasters that occurred between 1980 and 2004.

The Insurance Services Office (ISO) defines a catastrophe as an event that causes $24 million or more in insured property losses and affects a significant number of property/casualty policyholders and insurers. Catastrophe losses surged in 2008, reaching $25.2 billion, the highest since the record $62.5 billion reached in 2005,

Exhibit 1.5 Percentage of Businesses That Have Experienced Interruption

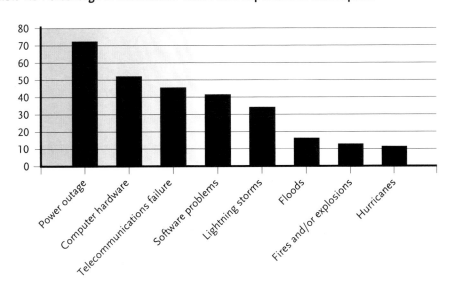

Source: Adapted from Baum and McDaniel (2008). Data from Zinkewicz (2005).

Exhibit 1.6 Disaster Toll, 1980 to 2004

Number of events	14,216
Deaths	1,049,006
Total property losses	$1,825 billion
Insured property losses	$374 billion

Source: Data from Munich Re (2010a).

Exhibit 1.7 Costliest Catastrophes in History

Month/Year	Peril	*Insured Loss (in billions of dollars)*	*2007 Dollars Loss (in billions of dollars)*
August 2005	Hurricane Katrina	$41.1*	$43.6
August 1992	Hurricane Andrew	$15.5	$22.9
September 2001	World Trade Center and Pentagon attacks	$18.8 (property claims only)	$22.0
January 1994	Earthquake in Northridge, California	$12.5	$17.5
October 2005	Hurricane Wilma	$10.3	$10.9
August 2004	Hurricane Charley	$7.5	$8.2
September 2004	Hurricane Ivan	$7.1	$7.8
September 1989	Hurricane Hugo	$4.2	$7.0
September 2005	Hurricane Rita	$5.6	$6.0
September 2004	Hurricane Frances	$4.6	$5.0

*The National Flood Insurance Program paid $15.6 billion in Katrina claims, in addition to the $40.6 billion paid by private insurers.

Source: ISO (2010).

the year of hurricanes Katrina and Rita and the fourth costliest year in a decade. There were 37 catastrophes in 2008, the highest number of catastrophic events in a year since 1998 (ISO 2010).

The catastrophe definition continually changes. ISO's (2010) Property Claim Services (PCS) revealed that from 1949 to 1982, a catastrophe was an event with a $1 million impact. From 1983 to 1996, the financial impact that defined an event as a catastrophe was $5 million. PCS now defines catastrophes as events that cause $25 million or more in direct insured losses to property and that affect a significant number of policyholders and insurers. And this number will most likely continue to increase. Exhibit 1.7 lists the costliest catastrophes that have occurred in the United States.

With 860 loss events due to natural hazards, the number of catastrophes documented in 2009 exceeded the previous year's 750 and the ten-year average of 770. The overall loss amounted to $50 billion, with 17 events exceeding the $1 billion threshold. The insurance industry incurred losses of $22 billion.

Of all natural catastrophes worldwide in 2009, 93 percent were caused by atmospheric conditions and 7 percent by earthquakes and volcanic eruptions. The breakdown by continent shows that most of the events occurred in the Americas and Asia (300 events and 290 events, respectively) compared with just under 130 in Europe and roughly 70 each in Australia and Africa (Munich Re 2010b).

HOSPITAL AWARENESS OF INCREASING DISASTERS

Although disasters are increasing in frequency and severity, the leading healthcare organizations in the United States often fail to treat this as a critical issue. The *2009 American Hospital Association Environmental Scan* "provides insight and information about market forces that have a high probability of affecting the health care field"; however, it does not mention emergencies, disasters, catastrophes, or any of the associated issues that have devastated hospitals and health delivery systems over the past decade. The most closely related item that made its list was advances in "vaccines for many infections that will be more effective and have fewer side effects." Widely acknowledged or not, preparedness for disaster response has increasingly become a priority for hospital leaders (Center for Biosecurity of UPMC 2009).

Vulnerability to Disasters

The trend toward increasing population densities and the progressive movement of these populations to disaster-prone flood plains, coastal regions at risk for hurricanes, areas with high seismic activity, and to communities constructed in areas vulnerable to wildland fires, means our potential for catastrophic disasters is increasing. (Auf der Heide 1996, 454)

Events since the 1980s and continuing threats have led to concerns about domestic terrorism. We have become more vulnerable to the risks posed by the manufacture, storage, and transportation of hazardous chemicals. Some of the largest civilian disasters in North America have been hazardous materials accidents.

Domestic civilian disasters are also characterized by a predominance of relatively low-severity injuries. "In a study of 29 U.S. major mass casualty incidents (MCIs), the Disaster Research Center found that less than 10 percent of the casualties had conditions that under ordinary circumstances would require overnight hospital admission. In actuality, about twice this number were admitted. For about half, it was more that they were involved in the disaster than because of the severity of their conditions" (Auf der Heide 1996, 455).

Preparedness

> The better prepared we are, the less likely we are to be traumatized when things go wrong and the quicker we can get back up on our feet and resume a normal life. (Flynn 2007)

Awareness of the risk of disasters is crucial, and preparing your organization and staff to function in these potential events is imperative.

Drs. Joe Barbera and Anthony MacIntyre are disaster experts and recognized leaders in this field. They write, "It is clear that hospital readiness remains uneven across the United States." Without significant disaster experience, many hospitals remain unprepared for natural disasters. They may be even less ready to accept the care for patient surge from chemical or biological attacks, conventional or nuclear explosive detonations, unusual natural disasters, or novel infectious disease outbreaks. The researchers report that the following factors promote hospital preparedness (Barbera, Yeatts, and MacIntyre 2009):

- Funding
- Federal government focus and guidance
- Standards and regulations
- Experience with and examples of adverse outcomes from inadequate preparation
- Community standards for involving and supporting local hospitals (increasing recognition of the importance of hospitals as critical infrastructure and emergency response assets)

Other factors are obstacles to adequate preparedness. Medical economics limits hospital motivation for funding preparedness. Most businesses in general fail to perceive the disaster risk, and the federal focus on preparing for unexpected events is foreign to them. The business and legal risks of preparedness are also an issue. Developing a common hazard vulnerability analysis (HVA) may be seen as perilous in that it divulges information related to operational strengths and vulnerabilities or other sensitive or proprietary information to rival organizations. Few legal precedents exist to establish clear answers to the many questions that arise. Finally, planning assumptions are based on conventional wisdom rather than on evidence or experience-based research. Hospitals expect an orderly distribution of casualties. They expect those casualties to be safe (noncontaminated) and to be transported by ambulance. And they expect prompt and comprehensive community service if the hospital is not compromised in any way, which is one of the most dangerous assumptions. However, in a disaster event, none of these assumptions is safe.

Cost Versus Benefit

Since their evolution from a social services model to a business model, hospitals are expected to operate using modern business efficiencies and cost justification. Despite this evolution, the public and policymakers expect that hospitals will be fully prepared for any hazard and provide needed medical services in the case of a disaster. Although many hospitals are private sector assets, they are expected during disasters to serve an essentially public sector function. They are also expected to function as key facilities and to maintain services in spite of direct hazard impact on their facilities.

The financial and personnel time cost associated with emergency preparedness can be a major disincentive. Hospital executives may feel that focusing on preparedness produces few tangible benefits. Many prefer to use insurance as protection, rather than emergency preparedness, especially for low-likelihood hazards. "Experienced executives recognize that poor response to disasters can create enterprise-level risk that is not covered by insurance [and] ethical dilemmas and permit compromise of professional reputations" (Barbera, Yeatts, and MacIntrye 2009).

The Hospital Preparedness Program (HPP)

In *Hospitals Rising to the Challenge: The First Five Years of the U.S. Hospital Preparedness Program and Priorities Going Forward* (Center for Biosecurity UPMC 2009), the assistant secretary for Preparedness and Response reports the following key findings:

- Disaster preparedness of individual hospitals has improved significantly throughout the country since the start of the Hospital Preparedness Program (HPP).
- The emergence of healthcare coalitions is creating a foundation of U.S. healthcare preparedness.

(continued)

- Healthcare planning for catastrophic emergencies is in its early stages; progress will require additional assistance and direction at the national level.
- Surge capacity and capability goals, assessment of training, and analysis of performance during actual events and realistic exercises are the most useful indicators for measuring preparedness.

Conclusions included the following:
- The HPP has improved the resilience of U.S. hospitals and communities and increased their capacity to respond to common medical disasters.
- The HPP should focus on building, strengthening, and linking healthcare coalitions to lay the foundation for a national disaster health and medical response system.
- Administrative adjustments to the HPP could improve the program's effectiveness and efficiency.
- To prepare the nation to respond to catastrophic emergencies, U.S. Department of Health and Human Services should provide continued leadership to states in their efforts to address the procedural, ethical, legal, and practical problems posed by a shift to disaster standards and alternate care facilities that is required when demand for care overwhelms available resources.
- Catastrophic emergency preparedness is a national security issue and requires the continued funding of the HPP.

> The U.S. healthcare system is not currently capable of effectively responding to a sudden surge in demand for medical care that would occur during catastrophic events, such as those described in the Department of Homeland Security's (DHS) National Planning Scenarios. Emergencies of this magnitude would overwhelm the medical capabilities of communities, regions, or the entire country and require drastic departures from customary healthcare practices. Such a "phase shift" in the provision of care to disaster standards would be unlike anything that has ever been done in the U.S. (Center for Biosecurity UPMC 2009)

> Prior to 2002, most hospitals did not have adequate plans to handle common medical disasters, much less catastrophic emergencies comparable to the National Planning Scenarios. Over the course of six years, the HPP has catalyzed significant improvements in hospital preparedness for common medical disasters. Hospitals have implemented communications systems, incident command system concepts, stockpiles of medicines and supplies, situational awareness tools, and memoranda of understanding (MOU) for sharing assets and staff during disasters. (Center for Biosecurity UPMC 2009)

> Risk perception may be negatively affected by the traditional hazard vulnerability analysis (HVA). The Joint Commission requires all hospitals and

healthcare organizations to conduct an HVA, which ranks hazards in their order of priority, rather than developing an understanding of vulnerability elements that are much more amenable to achieving risk reduction. Preparing only for Armageddon-level threats may result in a sense of futility or complete apathy. (Barbera, Yeatts, and MacIntyre 2009)

INCIDENT VERSUS EVENT

Are you preparing for an "incident" or an "event"? For the Oklahoma State Department of Health, these are two very different things (Ames 2009).

- An "incident" is any unplanned occurrence.
- An "event" is a planned occurrence.

Further confusing the terminology, the Department of Homeland Security (2008) states that an "incident"

- is an occurrence or event, natural or manmade, that requires a response to protect life or property
- and can include major disasters, emergencies, terrorist attacks, terrorist threats, civil unrest, wildland and urban fires, floods, hazardous materials spills, nuclear accidents, aircraft accidents, earthquakes, hurricanes, tornadoes, tropical storms, tsunamis, war-related disasters, public health and medical emergencies, and other occurrences requiring an emergency response.

Public Health Terminology

The public health profession uses terminology in a different manner. Again, using Oklahoma as an example, a "catastrophic health emergency" is an occurrence of imminent threat of an illness or health condition that (Oklahoma Legislature 2003)

- is believed to be caused by any of the following:
  - a nuclear attack
  - bioterrorism
  - a chemical attack, or
  - appearance of a novel or previously controlled or eradicated infectious agent or biological toxin; and

- poses a high probability of any of the following harms:
  - a large number of deaths in the affected population,
  - a large number of serious or long-term disabilities in the affected population, or
  - widespread exposure to an infectious or toxic agent that poses a significant risk of substantial future harm to a large number of people in the affected population.

An executive order of the governor will declare a "state of catastrophic health emergency," which activates disaster response and recovery aspects of the state, local, and interjurisdictional disaster emergency plans. During a state of emergency, the governor of Oklahoma may (Oklahoma Legislature 2003)

- suspend provisions of any regulatory statute prescribing procedures for conducting state business, orders, and rules of any state agency;
- use all available resources of state government and its political subdivisions;
- transfer direction, personnel, or functions of state departments and agencies to perform or facilitate response and recovery programs;
- mobilize all or part of the National Guard into services of the state;
- provide aid to and seek aid from other states (re interstate compact); and
- seek aid from the federal government.

Public health has primary jurisdiction over, responsibility for, and authority for

- planning and executing the catastrophic health emergency assessment, mitigation, preparedness, response, and recovery for the state;
- coordinating the catastrophic health emergency response between state and local authorities;
- collaborating with relevant federal government authorities, elected officials of other states, private organizations, or companies;
- coordinating recovery operations and mitigation initiatives; and
- organizing public information activities.

CHAPTER 2

Organizing for Disasters

The events of September 11, 2001, brought to light many gaps in our ability to prepare for, respond to, and recover from a major incident. They demonstrated the urgent need for national standards for incident operations, communications, personnel qualifications, resource and information management, and supporting technology. Communication equipment was not interoperable, and no one system could ensure preparedness, response, and recovery coordination and cooperation across all provider levels. Since that day, hospitals have faced new challenges to protect and care for their communities, especially in regard to the threat of bioterrorism.

In the United States, federal-level guidance and program development in disaster preparedness improvement has since soared. A number of crucial programs and documents guide comprehensive emergency management (CEM), which consists of the preparedness, response, recovery, and mitigative actions of healthcare providers. Exhibit 2.1 depicts these four phases of comprehensive emergency management.

All disasters are local. Response is progressive and can involve assistance from higher levels of the emergency management community. Once the resources of one level are expended, support from a higher level may be requested. Requests move from the local, to the county (or parish or burrough), to the state and federal levels, creating a layered response strategy.

Each level of response expands the healthcare organization's capabilities. An effective response requires participation from private entities, nongovernmental agencies, tribal or local jurisdiction government resources, state-level resources, and federal resources. Most incidents are resolved at the local or regional level, without the intervention or involvement of the federal government. If federal involvement is needed, it is focused on specific authorities or day-to-day functions, such as a hazardous materials response.

Exhibit 2.1 The Four Phases of Comprehensive Emergency Management, Plus Prevention

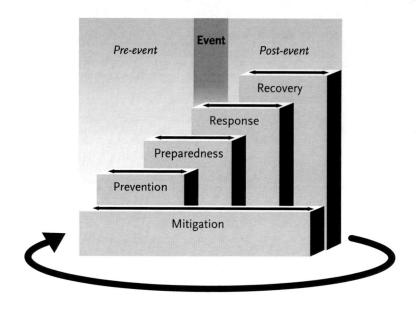

THE RESPONSE DOCTRINE

The goals of our national response doctrine are saving lives and protecting property and the environment. It is rooted in our federal system and the constitutional division of responsibilities between federal and state governments. It reflects the history of emergency management and the wisdom of responders and leaders at all levels and gives elemental form to the *National Response Framework* (NRF), or the *Framework*. The doctrine is made up of five key principles (DHS 2008, 8):

1. Engaged partnership
2. Tiered response
3. Scalable, flexible, and adaptable operational capabilities
4. Unity of effort through unified command
5. Readiness to act

The *Framework* sets out the roles and responsibilities of key implementers at the local, tribal, state, and federal levels. This includes the roles of private sector and nongovernmental organizations (NGOs) (DHS 2008, 15).

Dr. John Harrald (1998) of George Washington University describes public sector emergency management as having "the objectives of preserving the lives and social welfare and protecting the property of a defined population (city, county, state, country, region, etc.). Emergency management has typically been the province of government and not-for-profit organizations such a FEMA and the American Red Cross. These organizations exist because the population at risk requires their services: mitigation, preparation, response and recovery."

The Local Role

In that all disasters are local, response begins at the local level. Local leaders and emergency managers prepare their communities to manage incidents through the organization of resources and agencies in a spirit of cooperation, collaboration, coordination, and communication.

The local area may not have a designated emergency management agency (EMA) or an emergency operations center. Instead, these may be present only at the county level. However, an EMA structure and system exists to support healthcare delivery at each locality in a disaster. Each level of response brings an increased capability and additional personnel and resources to support a successful response.

The local area will stage the initial response to an event using local resources. If its resources are depleted or inadequate to respond to the event, it may request additional support from its county-level EMA. In a large event, multiple counties may be asked to respond. This request may be made to the county EMA director by the local EMA director, if there is one, or by the chief elected or appointed official (mayor or city or county manager). The local emergency manager has the day-to-day authority and responsibility for overseeing emergency management programs and activities.

The Four Cs of Successful Integration

Although these four items are important in every interaction and aspect of emergency management, it is imperative that they start at the local healthcare level.

1. Communication
Disasters require healthcare providers and entities to maintain open channels of communication with multiple entities to facilitate resource requests and deployment, emergency notifications, and situational updates. Different devices are available to assist

communications; however, they must be "multiple and redundant" and should allow providers to communicate in a planned manner with all agencies critical to the healthcare response. Exercises and drills should be conducted to test and improve communication plans and systems.

2. Cooperation

Healthcare organizations compete for patients and the services they require. In this competitive environment, information is carefully guarded. Healthcare providers deliver care to each individual, focusing on the health status of one person at a time.

Public health provides services to the general population. Health departments promote wellness and manage infectious diseases or unhealthy environmental conditions, among other responsibilities. Only since the advent of federal bio-terrorism preparedness programs in the past few years have health departments ventured beyond their usual scope of activities. Yet public health departments license healthcare facilities, and this creates a natural tension between these types of organizations.

Healthcare facilities and public service agencies, including EMAs, operate in different worlds. With the exception of emergency medical services (EMS), their respective activities have few natural intersections. Joint planning and preparedness activities, such as drills and exercises, can lower these barriers to cooperation.

3. Collaboration

Three activities promote and develop collaboration and better integrate the health-care community with its community partners in emergency preparedness and response: planning, training, and exercising.

Using a standard format for plans allows others to easily understand and coop-erate during the planning process, simplifying the sharing of information and exchange of knowledge. Planning together also helps each party understand the others' resources and capabilities. The most important outcome of collaborative planning is not the plan itself but the relationships that develop through the plan-ning process.

Training and performing disaster exercises together to test the plans are crucial to build relationships, strengthen response, and create an environment of trust and familiarity.

4. Coordination

Coordination is creating activities that are in harmony with the efforts of others. In a medical coordinating center, healthcare facilities and public health agencies can work together to coordinate management of the health effects of a major incident.

And the Joint Information Center can provide a single voice to send a message to the public or to all participating agencies and organizations.

Local-level partners in strengthening the healthcare response may include:

- Public safety: local police or sheriff, fire services and hazmat, EMS
- Education: local school districts, universities and community colleges, vocational and technical schools
- Transportation: city and county department of transportation; city airports
- Human services: welfare and homeless services, social services agencies, mental health/counseling services
- Health resources: local public health departments, local environmental protection agencies
- Infrastructure: city utility companies (water, power, sewer), public works
- Local media outlets

The State Role

The primary role of state government is to supplement and facilitate local efforts before, during, and after incidents. Thus, the role of the state EMA is to assist local areas and agencies in all activities related to CEM.

At the local and state levels, EMAs play a critical role in supporting the response to any major incident or disaster. States provide resources and support to responses at the local and county level. When state resources are scarce or when the event exceeds the state's ability to respond appropriately, the governor may make a formal request of the president for federal assistance. This occurs through the granting of one of two types of presidential disaster declarations.

State-level partners of interest to healthcare providers may include:

- The state Homeland Security advisor
- The director of the state EMA
- State departments and agencies
- Indian tribal leaders
- Public safety: state police or patrol, the state fire marshal, the state EMS agency
- Education: universities and community colleges, vocational and technical schools
- Transportation: the department of transportation, the highway and roads department, aviation administrations
- Human services: welfare and social services agencies, mental health/counseling services, labor services

- Health resources: state health departments, environmental agencies, the radiation regulatory agency
- Infrastructure: utility companies (water, power, sewer), communications companies (telephone, Internet)

Federal Direction

The president leads the federal government response effort to ensure that the necessary coordinating structures, leadership, and resources are applied quickly and efficiently to large-scale and catastrophic incidents. Through the Homeland Security Council and the National Security Council, Cabinet officers and other department or agency heads provide national strategic and policy advice to the president (DHS 2008, 24). When state resources are depleted or inadequate to stage an effective response to a disaster, the governor may make a formal request of the president for a federal declaration of disaster. This declaration is beneficial in a large-scale incident, as it provides access to federal resources and initiates federal disaster reimbursement mechanisms.

Exhibit 2.2 Bottom-Up Response

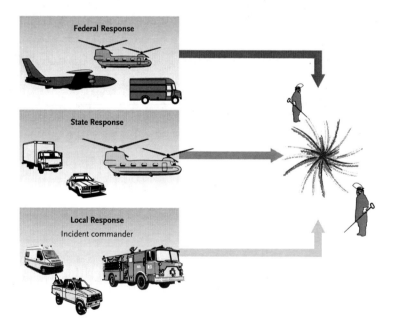

Exhibit 2.2 illustrates the "bottom up" response to a local incident, with resources and assistance starting at the local level and supported with a state response and, if warranted, a federal response.

Who's in Charge? Federal Declaration of Disaster or Public Health Emergency

The Pandemic and All-Hazards Preparedness Act of 2006 (P.L. 109-417) designates the secretary of the Department of Health and Human Services (HHS) as the lead for all federal public health and medical responses to public health emergencies and incidents covered by the National Response Plan (NRP) or its successor, the National Response Framework (NRF). The HHS assistant secretary for preparedness and response (ASPR) is the secretary's principal advisor on matters related to federal public health and medical preparedness and response for public health emergencies.

Under the NRF, HHS is the lead agency for Emergency Support Function (ESF) 8, the Public Health and Medical Services Annex, and the Biological Incident Annex. HHS also plays a significant role as a supporting agency for ESF 6, the Mass Care, Housing, and Human Services Annex.

What's an 1135 Waiver?

Section 143 of the Public Health Security and Bioterrorism Preparedness and Response Act of 2002 authorizes the HHS secretary to temporarily waive or modify Medicare, Medicaid, and Children's Health Insurance Program (CHIP) requirements when the president declares an emergency or major disaster pursuant to the Stafford Act or the National Emergencies Act and the HHS secretary declares a public health emergency.

Certain Program Requirements That May Be Waived (abbreviated)

- Conditions of participation
- Pre-approval requirements for providers or for healthcare items or services
- Requirements that physicians and other healthcare professionals hold licenses in the state in which they provide services
- Sanctions under EMTALA for redirection of an individual to another location to receive a medical screening examination pursuant to a state emergency preparedness plan
- Sanctions related to Stark self-referral prohibitions
- Deadlines and timetables for performance of required activities
- Limitations on payments to permit Medicare Advantage enrollees to use out-of-network providers in an emergency situation
- Sanctions and penalties arising from noncompliance with HIPAA privacy regulations, in 3 areas, for a 72-hour period after a hospital implements its disaster protocol

Source: Ray (2009, 254)

The Federal Declaration of Disaster or Public Health Emergency

During a public health or other emergency, the ability of a government official to declare an emergency can be an important tool from a legal perspective. While HHS has broad authority to assist states and other entities during an emergency, even without a public health emergency (PHE) declaration, such a declaration can facilitate HHS's preparation and mobilization by authorizing the secretary to take certain actions to respond to the emergency. It may allow officials to exercise special powers and permit them to suspend certain legal requirements to respond to the event.

Two types of disaster declarations may be made at the federal level:

1. A presidential declaration of an emergency or major disaster, under the Robert T. Stafford Disaster Relief and Emergency Assistance Act (Stafford Act), which usually requires a formal request by a state governor
2. A Public Health Emergency (PHE) declaration, which the HHS secretary may declare under Section 319 of the Public Health Service (PHS) Act without a formal request from a governor or other entity

THE NATIONAL STRATEGY FOR HOMELAND SECURITY: THE FRAMEWORK, THE GOAL, AND HSPDS

Recognizing the inherent weaknesses caused by inadequate and uncoordinated emergency systems, the president issued two directives that resulted in our national strategy for Homeland Security, Homeland Security Presidential Directives (HSPDs) 5 and 8, mandating the development of a fully integrated and interoperable planning and response system. Exhibit 2.3 illustrates the National Strategy for Homeland Security. It presents the related HSPDs and the national initiatives that complement them.

HSPD-5 mandated the establishment of a single, comprehensive system to manage incidents, the National Incident Management System (NIMS), while HSPD -8 required a national domestic all-hazards preparedness goal with mechanisms for improved delivery of federal preparedness assistance to state and local governments (Bush 2003).

HSPD-5

HSPD-5 institutionalized the all-hazards approach and promoted full integration of all phases of incident management. It included the NRP and NIMS (Hess 2004).

Exhibit 2.3 National Strategy for Homeland Security

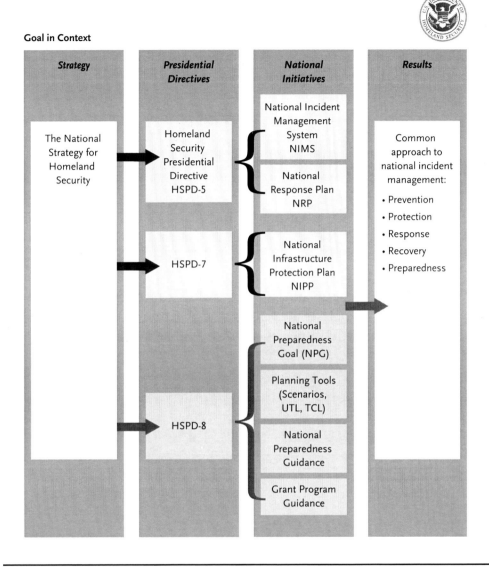

The NRP, using the NIMS, provides structure and mechanisms for national-level policy and operational direction for federal support to state and local incident managers, and for exercising direct federal authorities and responsibilities. Other objectives were to (Hess 2004):

◆ ensure a system that allows all levels of government to work efficiently and effectively together,
◆ provide seamless integration of resources and capabilities,

- provide a common lexicon and systems for horizontal and vertical integration,
- establish networks and systems for effective communication,
- ensure full integration of the crisis and consequence management components of incident management, and
- eliminate any barriers between the criminal investigation and emergency response components in a terrorism event.

HSPD-5 designates the secretary of Homeland Security as the principal federal official for domestic incident management. In catastrophic events, the secretary may designate a principal federal official (PFO) as his or her representative. The PFO provides senior leadership for the event but does not replace or duplicate the roles of other emergency managers.

HSPD-8

On December 17, 2003, the president issued HSPD-8. A companion to HSPD-5, this directive establishes policies to strengthen the nation's preparedness to prevent and respond to threatened or actual domestic terrorist attacks, major disasters, and other emergencies by

- requiring a national domestic all-hazards preparedness goal,
- establishing mechanisms for improved delivery of federal preparedness assistance to state and local governments, and
- outlining actions to strengthen the preparedness capabilities of federal, state, and local entities.

NATIONAL PREPAREDNESS GUIDELINES AND STRATEGY

The national strategy for Homeland Security uses a capabilities-based planning approach: planning, under uncertainty, to provide capabilities suitable for a wide range of threats and hazards within an economic framework that necessitates prioritization and choice (DHS 2010). The strategy states that our nation should focus its efforts on four goals:

1. Prevent and disrupt terrorist attacks.
2. Protect the American people, our critical infrastructure, and key resources.
3. Respond to and recover from incidents.

4. Continue to strengthen the emergency-preparedness foundation.

By 2005, planning tools had become available to assist in implementation of the national preparedness goal (NPG). Using 15 national planning scenarios of plausible catastrophic terrorist attacks, major disasters, and other emergencies, a universal task list (UTL) provides a menu of tasks from all sources that may be performed in major events. The target capabilities list (TCL) provides guidance on specific capabilities and levels of capability that federal, state, local, and tribal entities will be expected to develop and maintain.

NATIONAL INCIDENT MANAGEMENT SYSTEM (NIMS)

NIMS is a companion document to the NRP, superceded by the NRF. It provides standard command and management structures that apply to response activities and a consistent nationwide template to enable all government, private sector, and nongovernmental organizations to work together during domestic incidents. NIMS provides the common operational concepts and basic organizational structure to ensure seamless transitions and integration of resources. This compatibility and interoperability is critical, especially in incidents that exceed local boundaries. The organizational structure ensures that responders from anywhere in the nation can work together, regardless of the nature or the location of the incident. Responders know where they fit into the organization, they know their own roles and responsibilities, and they know what is expected of them.

Components of NIMS for Hospitals and Healthcare Systems

NIMS is built in a flexible framework around five key components:

1. Adoption of NIMS
2. Planning
3. Training and exercises
4. Communications and information management
5. Command and management

The *NIMS Implementation Activities for Hospitals and Healthcare Systems* (FEMA 2006) lists 14 activities related to these five components that must be completed for hospitals and healthcare systems to comply with NIMS.

Exhibit 2.4 NIMS Implementation Activities

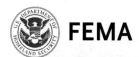 **FEMA**

FY 2008 NIMS Compliance Objectives

Adoption

1. Adopt NIMS throughout the healthcare organization, including all appropriate departments and business units.
2. Ensure Federal Preparedness awards support NIMS Implementation (in accordance with the eligibility and allowable uses of the awards).

Preparedness: Planning

3. Revise and update emergency operations plans (EOPs), standard operating procedures (SOPs), and standard operating guidelines (SOGs) to incorporate NIMS and National Response Framework (NRF) components, principles, and policies, to include planning, training, response, exercises, equipment, evaluation, and corrective actions.
4. Participate in interagency mutual aid and/or assistance agreements, to include agreements with public and private sector and nongovernmental organizations.

Preparedness: Training and Exercises

5. Identify the appropriate personnel to complete ICS-100, ICS-200, and IS-700, or equivalent courses.
6. Identify the appropriate personnel to complete IS-800 or an equivalent course.
7. Promote NIMS concepts and principles into all organization-related training and exercises. Demonstrate the use of NIMS principles and ICS Management structure in training and exercises.

Communications and Information Management

8. Promote and ensure that equipment, communication, and data interoperability are incorporated into the healthcare organization's acquisition programs.
9. Apply common and consistent terminology as promoted in NIMS, including the establishment of plain language communications standards.
10. Utilize systems, tools, and processes that facilitate the collection and distribution of consistent and accurate information during an incident or event.

Command and Management

11. Manage all emergency incidents, exercises, and preplanned (recurring/special) events in accordance with ICS organizational structures, doctrine, and procedures, as defined in NIMS.
12. ICS implementation must include the consistent application of Incident Action Planning (IAP) and common communications plans, as appropriate.
13. Adopt the principle of Public Information, facilitated by the use of the Joint Information System (JIS) and Joint Information Center (JIC) during an incident or event.
14. Ensure that Public Information procedures and processes gather, verify, coordinate, and disseminate information during an incident or event.

Hospitals are not mandated to comply, but they will not receive certain federal funding if they do not. The National Bioterrorism Hospital Preparedness Program of the HHS assistant secretary for preparedness and response (ASPR) to the state's department of health has provided implementation guidance and deadlines. The current 14 implementation activities are consistent with the NIMS components. Exhibit 2.4 illustrates the 14 implementation activities for hospital compliance.

THE NATIONAL RESPONSE FRAMEWORK (NRF)

The NRF replaces the NRP. NRF provides guiding principles for a unified national response. It is built on a scalable, flexible, and adaptable coordinating structure to align key roles and responsibilities across the nation. It describes specific authorities and best practices for managing incidents that range from the serious but purely local to large-scale terrorist attacks or catastrophic natural disasters. Most important, it builds upon NIMS, which provides a consistent template for managing incidents (DHS 2008, 1).

The National Response Framework (NRF)
The Framework is made up of the core document, the Emergency Support Functions (ESF), Support and Incident Annexes, and the Partner Guides.

- The Core Document lays out the doctrine that guides our national response, explains the roles and responsibilities of the individuals and organizations involved, presents the response actions that should be taken, and lists the response organizations and planning requirements needed to achieve an effective national response to any incident.
- Emergency Support Function (ESF) Annexes group federal resources and capabilities into the functional areas that are most frequently needed in a national response.
- Support Annexes describe essential supporting aspects that are common to all incidents, such as financial management and private sector coordination.
- Incident Annexes address unique aspects of our responses to seven broad incident categories (e.g., mass evacuation, biological, cyber).

THE CATASTROPHIC INCIDENT SUPPLEMENT (CIS) TO THE CATASTROPHIC INCIDENT ANNEX TO THE NATIONAL RESPONSE FRAMEWORK (NRF-CIS)

A *catastrophic incident*, as defined by the National Response Framework, is any natural or man-made incident, including terrorism, that results in extraordinary levels of mass casualties, damage, or disruption severely affecting the population, infrastructure, environment, economy, national morale, and/or government functions. A catastrophic incident could result in sustained nationwide impacts over a prolonged period of time; almost immediately exceeds resources normally available to state, tribal, local, and private-sector authorities in the impacted area; and significantly interrupts governmental operations and emergency services to such an extent that national security could be threatened. These factors drive the urgency for coordinated national planning to ensure accelerated federal and/or national assistance (DHS 2008).

A catastrophic incident will likely trigger a presidential major disaster declaration. In these situations, the National Response Framework Catastrophic Incident Annex (CIA) is designed to address (DHS 2008)

1. no-notice or short-notice incidents of catastrophic magnitude,
2. where the need for Federal assistance is obvious and immediate,
3. where anticipatory planning and resource pre-positioning were precluded, and
4. where the exact nature of needed resources and assets is not known.

The planning assumption is that a catastrophic incident will result in many casualties and displaced persons, possibly in the tens to hundreds of thousands. In an incident response, human life–saving operations are given priority.

INCIDENT CONDITIONS

Normal procedures for certain emergency support functions may be expedited or streamlined to address the magnitude of the incident. The federal government and other national entities will provide expedited assistance in one or more of the following areas:

- Mass Evacuations (ESF #5)
- Mass Care, Housing, and Human Services (ESF #6)
- Search and Rescue (ESF #9)
- Victim Decontamination (ESF #8) or Environmental Assessment and Decontamination (ESF #10)

- Public Health and Medical Support (ESF #8)
- Medical Equipment and Supplies (ESF #8)
- Casualty Transportation (ESF #8)
- Public Safety and Security (ESF #13)
- Public Information (ESF #15)
- Critical Infrastructure Support

The Emergency Support Functions of the NRF

The federal resources of the NRF are organized along 15 ESFs. Each has a designated co-ordination agency, which is supported by resources from across the entire array of federal agencies and resources. The ESFs and their primary federal coordinating agency are:

ESF #1: Transportation (DOT)
ESF #2: Communications (DHS/National Communications System)
ESF #3: Public Works and Engineering (DOD/U.S. Army Corps of Engineers)
ESF #4: Firefighting (U.S. Department of Agriculture)
ESF #5: Emergency Management (DHS/FEMA)
ESF #6: Mass Care, Housing, and Human Services (DHS/FEMA)
ESF #7: Resource Support (GSA)
ESF #8: Public Health and Medical Services (HHS)
ESF #9: Urban Search and Rescue (DHS/FEMA)
ESF #10: Oil and Hazardous Materials Response (EPA)
ESF #11: Agriculture and Natural Resources (U.S. Department of Agriculture)
ESF #12: Energy (DOE)
ESF #13: Public Safety and Security (DOJ)
ESF #14: Long-Term Community Recovery (DHS/FEMA)
ESF #15: External Affairs (DHS)

Health and medical functions fall primarily under ESF#8, Public Health and Medical Services, and ESF#6, Mass Care, Housing, and Human Services. HHS is the lead federal agency for ESF#8, with operational control of the U.S. Public Health Service. HHS also plays a significant role as a supporting agency for ESF#6, with FEMA as the lead federal agency.

REGULATORY AND STANDARDS-SETTING AGENCIES

A plethora of federal agencies provide input into the regulation and guidance of healthcare preparation for and response to disasters and critical events. The following is a list of agency categories and examples of each.

- Regulatory: Occupational Safety and Health Administration, Centers for Medicare & Medicaid Services
- Nonregulatory: Centers for Disease Control and Prevention (CDC), Office of the Assistant Secretary for Preparedness and Response, Agency for Healthcare Research and Quality, FEMA's Incident Management Systems Division
- Accrediting: The Joint Commission, Community Health Accreditation Program, American Osteopathic Association
- Standards setting: National Fire Protection Agency (NFPA), American Institute of Architects
- Professional Organizations: American College of Healthcare Executives (ACHE), American Hospital Association, American Public Health Association

The Federal Response Process

Guiding principles for a proactive federal catastrophic incident response include the following.

- The primary mission is to save lives, protect property and critical infrastructure, contain the event, and protect the national security.
- Standard procedures may be expedited or temporarily suspended in the immediate aftermath of a catastrophic magnitude event.
- Pre-identified federal resources are mobilized and deployed.
- Notification and full coordination with states occur, but the rapid mobilization and deployment of critical federal resources should not be delayed by the coordination process.
- The secretary of Homeland Security immediately begins implementation of the NRF-CIA. Federal departments and agencies immediately
  - take actions to activate, mobilize, and deploy incident-specific resources in accordance with the NRF-CIS;
  - take actions to protect life, property, and critical infrastructure under their jurisdiction and provide assistance within the affected area;
  - commence those hazard-specific activities established under the appropriate and applicable NRF Incident Annexes, including the NRF-CIA; and
  - commence those functional activities and responsibilities established under the NRF ESF Annexes.

Based on notice and time for coordination and assessment, NRF-CIA actions that the federal government may take in response to a catastrophic incident may include

- mobilization and deployment of resources by scenario type;
- predeployment of appropriately tailored elements specified in the NRF-CIS, to meet the anticipated demands of the specific incident scenario; or

- provision of DOD capabilities in the following support categories: aviation, communication, defense coordinating officer/element, medical treatment, patient evacuation, decontamination, and logistics.

Appendix 2.1: Using the Hazards and Vulnerability Analysis

1. A hazards and vulnerability analysis (HVA) is used to determine the hazards that pose a realistic risk of interrupting continuity of patient care services and demand for care, and other consequences of a disaster.
2. The HVA is a fundamental component of a comprehensive emergency management program and is a compliance requirement among many licensing and accreditation organizations.
3. Hazard-specific risks are determined by comparing the likelihood of an event occurring, the potential impacts to the organization, and mitigation activities that would be deployed. It is completed using input from clinical and nonclinical disciplines.
4. By prioritizing hazards, an organization is able to strategically fund appropriate mitigation activities. This is particularly prudent considering the competing resource priorities of more direct patient care–related programs.
5. Hazard-specific response plans will guide healthcare responders with precise, event-related activities.
6. Response guides should include how an incident is assessed; trigger points for response activation; recommendations of who should be mobilized; and specific actions, resources, and equipment needed for the response.
7. Response guides should be routinely tested, evaluated, modified, and re-tested to ensure high levels of organizational response competency.
8. The HVA should be evaluated annually and following each exercise or actual incident.
9. The HVA priorities and planning activities should be shared with community response agencies to improve overall regional response capability.
10. In most cases, the HVA, combined with measurable mitigation activities, can reduce organizational costs such as insurance requirements or recovery costs.

Source:
Mitch Saruwatari
Vice President, Quality and Compliance
LiveProcess, Inc.
October 2009

Appendix 2.2: Ethics in Healthcare Management

- Discuss how your organization would approach ethical issues in a disaster **before** the disaster occurs. Crisis situations are not the time to have philosophical discussions about belief systems, cultural issues, or altering your standard of care. These ethical conversations need to happen in a thoughtful, reflective environment, where all parties potentially involved in the outcome can provide input.

- Know your legal landscape. Know what laws and standards related to disaster management apply to your facility and your response to a situation. Who has authority in a disaster to make ethical and legal decisions? Have those people been participants in discussions about issues related to disasters? Do you know what are considered "acceptable exceptions" to patient care in a disaster? For example, when is it permissible to deviate from EMTALA or HIPAA regulations? Develop and maintain a list of resources for legal assistance and information and put it in your disaster response handbook.

- What planning have you done to expand your scope of services in a disaster beyond medical surge planning? Have you considered extending the scope of services for some of your staff? How you will manage volunteers coming into your facility? Will you alter your facility to accommodate patients beyond your bed capacity? Have you discussed how you would alter your standards of care (such as universal precautions) in a disaster?

- Play the game "Worst Case Scenario" for your agency or facility. Have some hard conversations about the worst situations you can imagine and discuss how you would manage those situations from an ethical standpoint. What if there were an epidemic and you had to decide who got treatment and who would be left to die?

- Don't assume! Do not assume that someone else will be making ethical legal decisions in a disaster. You never know what situation you may face. Hurricane Katrina taught us that lesson. The established lines of authority may not exist—you may be the only authority!

- What planning have you or your healthcare partners in the community done for vulnerable populations in a disaster? Special needs populations will have different and specialized needs in a crisis and will require more of your resources. How have you planned for these individuals? What ethical dilemmas would their care create?

- Identify resources. Know where you are going to get scarce resources. Have mutual aid agreements in hand with other healthcare facilities and with vendors so you have backup planning when the expected resources are not available or run out. This will avoid having to make ethical decisions as to who will get resources and who will not.

- Talk with your staff about ethical issues in disasters. What do they think their obligations are in a disaster? Should they be required to risk their lives? Would they choose their family over work, and if so, how can you help them to be better prepared at home for a disaster so they can report to work?

- Include ethical issues in your training exercises. Present your team with potential situations that make them consider what ethical decisions they may have to make.

- Know thyself! Examine your own cultural, religious, and life experiences and think about how you would react and make ethical decisions in a disaster. Again, the first time to have this conversation is not during the crisis, when decision-making skills and stress management are at their lowest level.

Source:
Dee Grimm, RN, JD
CEO
Emergency Management Professionals

CHAPTER 3

Preparedness Planning for Catastrophic Health Events

Let's talk about the realities. You can't be making this up in the throes of a disaster. —Phil Robinson

CATASTROPHIC HEALTH EVENTS (CHE)

As Homeland Security Presidential Directive 21 (HSPD-21) defines it, a CHE is "any natural or manmade incident, including terrorism, that results in a number of ill or injured persons sufficient to overwhelm the capabilities of immediate local and regional emergency response and health care systems" (DHS 2007).

> A catastrophic health event, such as a terrorist attack with a weapon of mass destruction (WMD), a naturally occurring pandemic, or a calamitous meteorological or geological event, could cause tens or hundreds of thousands of casualties or more, weaken our economy, damage public morale and confidence, and threaten our national security. It is therefore critical that we establish a strategic vision that will enable a level of public health and medical preparedness sufficient to address a range of possible disasters. (DHS 2007)

Planning Assumptions for Catastrophic Events
A catastrophic incident

- will result in a large number of casualties and/or displaced persons, possibly in the tens to hundreds of thousands;
- mandates giving priority to human life–saving operations (CAT-4);

(continued)

- will immediately overwhelm state, tribal, and local response capabilities and require immediate federal support;
- may delay a detailed and credible evaluation of the situation for 24 to 48 hours (or longer) after an incident, meaning response activities may have to begin without the benefit of a complete situation and critical needs assessment;
- has unique dimensions/characteristics that require response plans and strategies flexible enough to effectively address emerging needs;
- may occur with little or no warning and may be well underway before it is even detected;
- may be made up of multiple incidents occurring simultaneously or sequentially in contiguous and/or noncontiguous areas (some incidents, such as a biological WMD attack, may be dispersed over a large geographic area and lack a defined incident site);
- will produce environmental impacts that severely challenge the ability and capacity of governments and communities to achieve a timely recovery;
- may require federal resources capable of mobilization and deployment before they are requested via normal protocols;
- may result in organized or self-directed large-scale evacuations;
- may quickly overwhelm existing healthcare systems, requiring the evacuation of existing patients to accommodate increased patient workload if the facility remains operational (persons with special needs, including residents of nursing homes and extended care facilities, will require special attention during evacuation);
- may leave large numbers of people temporarily or permanently homeless (some displaced people will require specialized attention, healthcare assistance, and more); and
- will have significant international dimensions, including impacts on the health and welfare of border community populations, cross-border trade, transit, and law enforcement coordination.

Source: FEMA (2008)

ACHE Policy Statement: Healthcare Executives' Role in Emergency Preparedness
"As a critical component of a community's infrastructure, healthcare organizations should require proper planning for all-hazards events they may face. Healthcare executives should be active leaders in that planning and the creation of systems and processes to ensure that the emergency operating plan can be effectively and efficiently executed if ever needed" (ACHE 2009).
The American College of Healthcare Executives believes:

- healthcare executives should actively participate in disaster planning and preparedness activities;

- the CEO should lead efforts to ensure that the plan is comprehensive, including establishing board policy that delineates the organization's responsibilities and procedures to be followed; and
- the comprehensive emergency operations plan should include pursuing the following actions on an ongoing basis:
  - Maintain a relevant/current emergency or disaster plan that reflects current state and national standards for emergency preparedness, including the National Response Framework and the Hospital Preparedness Program
  - Focus the plan to address the most likely scenarios in an all-hazards framework
  - Develop an incident command system (ICS)
  - Assess resource availability
  - Plan for continuity of operations
  - Develop protocols to ensure appropriate resource allocation
  - Address the safety of employees, patients, and families
  - Design appropriate communication and coordination protocols for internal and external audiences
  - Enhance disease surveillance and reporting

ISSUES OF CATASTROPHIC DISASTER PREPAREDNESS AND PLANNING

While much progress has been made in healthcare preparedness for common medical disasters, the U.S. healthcare system is ill-prepared for catastrophic health events (CHE), and there is yet no clear strategy that will enable an effective response to such an event. (UPMC 2010a, i)

In a catastrophic health event, tens or hundreds of thousands of sick or injured individuals needing access to limited healthcare resources will quickly overwhelm local and extended systems. The goal of disaster planning for catastrophic events is to "surge" our capabilities and capacity far beyond what exists for day-to-day operations. This requires extensive thought, preparation, and planning long before a severe incident occurs.

When we speak of surge capacity, we are really talking about the ability to expand in four areas—the "four Ss of surge capacity" (Barbisch and Koenig 2006):

1. Staff: the human resources required to stage a response and sustain it
2. Stuff: the items and materials needed to provide a healthcare response
3. Structure: the physical facilities required to accommodate and deliver care for large volumes of patients

4. Strategy: the beneficial effect of preplanning an approach to an event

Accredited hospitals in the United States are required to have disaster plans and ensure that their employees are familiar with them. Yet, in many recent disasters hospitals were inadequately prepared for the substantive problems that developed. And although most hospitals have a written disaster plan, it is not necessarily accompanied by an adequate training program. This "paper plan syndrome" merely presents an illusion of preparedness (Auf der Heide 1989).

A disaster plan is only as effective as the assumptions on which it is based. Unfortunately, empirical studies have revealed that much of the conventional wisdom on which these plans have been based is incorrect (Auf der Heide 1996). For instance, medical disaster planning was traditionally based on a belief that the primary need in disasters is for large-scale mobilization of resources. This is based on the perception of disasters as emergencies that exceed the resources available to manage them. We now know this to be incorrect. In the United States, a shortage of resources is rare; however, problems arise when these resources are improperly managed.

The occurrence or threat of multiple or successive catastrophic incidents may significantly reduce the size, speed, and depth of the federal response. When deemed necessary or prudent, the federal government may reduce the allocation of finite resources for which multiple venues are competing (FEMA 2008). Thus, the collaborative nature of disaster response encourages states to work together and with the federal government in planning for catastrophic incidents.

All-Hazards Versus Scenario-Based Planning

The basic concept of all-hazards planning is that responses to disasters are the same, irrespective of the cause. This is the FEMA-supported methodology for disaster response planning. On the other hand, scenario-based planning uses a specific scenario to establish a framework for modeling disaster effects and potential needed resources and evaluating regional emergency management capabilities. This method uses decision matrices to quickly determine baseline estimates for resource needs and to identify possible shortfalls for various events. The entire emergency management system can easily be analyzed for gaps.

"When a disaster reaches catastrophic proportions, covering many jurisdictions, dissimilar response plans may make it difficult to conduct a coordinated response. Multijurisdictional, scenario-specific catastrophe response planning can significantly decrease the conflicts and inefficiencies that would otherwise exist" (Ruback, Wells, and Bissell 2009, 5).

Collaboration is required for a successful emergency response, and that collaboration must include planning, training, and exercises. Each of these occur internally (within each healthcare organization) and externally (in concert with community responders and based on higher-level guidance).

Many different types of plans are needed for a solid emergency management program. A tiered response to planning includes:

1. Personal and family preparedness
2. Departmental plans
3. Organizational plans
4. Community and regional plans
5. Statewide plans
6. Multistate and national plans

The healthcare organization should include the first three in its internal planning. The organizational planning should fit with the community and regional plans and should provide input into support of statewide planning efforts, should a catastrophic event occur.

Plans are developed for all four phases of comprehensive emergency management (CEM), but the two primary categories are preparedness and response. Preparedness plans include resource management, training and education, and exercise and evaluation plans. Response plans include the emergency operations plan (EOP) and business continuity plans (BCPs).

The VA's Nine Step Emergency Management Planning Process
Internally, the VA's Nine Step Emergency Management Planning Process is among the most rational and easily executed systems for building a strong level of internal preparedness that fully integrates with the community. The steps are illustrated below.

Step One: Form an Emergency Management Committee
1. The CEO appoints a chairperson—preferably the emergency manager—and committee members representing key hospital incident command system (HICS) functional areas and interested stakeholders.
2. The committee establishes regular meeting times.
3. The committee determines goals, milestones, and tasks.
4. The committee records meeting minutes to share with staff and brief management and board as appropriate.

(continued)

Step Two: Develop a Hazard Vulnerability Analysis (HVA)

1. This analysis can be personalized to determine the organization's vulnerability in specific areas, such as hazardous materials accidents and terrorism.
2. The analysis assesses probability, human impact, property impact, and operational impact.
3. There is no one required HVA template or tool. One excellent tool is an Excel-based spreadsheet developed for Kaiser Permanente and praised by FEMA for its ease of use (this is available at www.nhja.com [type "HVA" in the search field]).
4. Don't reinvent the wheel. Examine existing HVAs from your local or area EMA, and plan for the most likely and highest risk events.

Step Three: Develop Standard Operating Procedures (SOPs)

1. An SOP describes the threat or event and its impact on the mission, examines critical systems and operating units, and identifies key personnel with responsibility to manage the threat or event.
2. SOPs should be based on HVA results.
3. SOPs should include strategies addressing the four CEM phases: mitigation, preparedness, response, and recovery.
4. For mitigation and preparedness, SOPs should state several objectives or strategies for
   a. hazard reduction and resource issues and
   b. preparedness and resource issues.
5. For response and recovery from the event, SOPs should state several objectives or strategies for
   a. hazard control and resource issues,
   b. hazard monitoring, and
   c. recovery.
6. SOPs should list notification procedures for people within the facility and outside.
7. SOPs should identify specialized staff training, references, and further assistance (such as texts and manuals) to better prepare responders.

Step Four: Implement Mitigation and Preparedness Activities

1. Mitigation actions should be implemented to prevent or reduce the impact of structural and nonstructural hazards (e.g., building repairs, utility checks, safety standards, redundant communications, and security procedures).
2. Preparedness actions designed to build capacity, such as developing training programs, inventorying supplies, and formalizing agreements, should be implemented.

Step Five: Report Results of Mitigation and Preparedness to Emergency Management Committee

1. The EM committee should monitor and direct these activities.
2. The committee should routinely brief and update management.
3. The committee should recommend improvements to the EM program.

Step Six: Develop an Emergency Operations Plan
1. Incident command system/hospital incident command system (ICS/HICS) concepts should be applied throughout the plan.
2. The EOP should focus on response and the early stages of the recovery phase.
3. The EOP should include a base plan that describes operations (the organization's mission and actions during response and recovery) and systems (the organization of assets during response and recovery).
   a. EOP base plan: purpose, scope, policies, situation, planning assumptions, and concept of operations
   b. EOP functional annexes: procedures and guidance aligned with HICS functional areas (management, planning, operations, logistics, and finance).
   c. Attachments to functional annexes: may include checklists and guidance documentation, such as a mobilization checklist, a call-back roster, or job action sheets (JASs).

Step Seven: Conduct Staff Education and Training
1. All staff should be trained on potential roles in competency-based emergency management. They should also be familiar with the EOP, location of procedures, and activation processes.
2. Those expected to perform with HICS or in the command center should take the following courses: IS 100, 200, 700, and 800 (DHS 2008).
3. These and other training materials can be accessed at www.fema.gov or through local and state departments of health and emergency management agencies.

Step Eight: Implement or Exercise the Emergency Operations Plan and Conduct a Critique
1. Exercise the plan or experience an actual event. A successful exercise includes an assessment of need.
   a. Review the HVA.
   b. Review regulatory guidance.
   c. Assess past after-action reviews (AARs).
   d. Evaluate external involvement needs.
   e. Conduct an EOP review.
   f. Establish measurable criteria against which to conduct the exercise.
   g. Conduct an AAR to identify areas in need of change.

Step Nine: Annual Evaluation and Corrective Actions
1. Review and refine the emergency management plan (EMP).
2. Address exercise or actual-event AARs, training programs, competencies, HVA, SOPs, EOPs, interface with community and external agencies, formal agreements, staff roles, and healthcare mission and roles.

Crisis Standards of Care

During a catastrophic event, resources will likely be severely limited. Resource shortfalls may require rationing, which will affect the standards of care provided. A change from normal standards to crisis standards of care may be necessary. It is important to have a plan to address the legal, ethical, and emotional complexity of such issues prior to an event.

In September 2009, the Institute of Medicine (IOM 2009) released a study providing guidance to state and local public health officials in establishing and implementing standards of care that should apply in disaster situations when resources are scarce. These "crisis standards of care" must be consistent within the state and must be developed through collaboration with neighboring states and partners.

'Crisis standards of care' is defined as a substantial change in usual health care operations and the level of care it is possible to deliver, which is made necessary by a pervasive (e.g., pandemic influenza) or catastrophic (e.g., earthquake, hurricane) disaster. This change in the level of care delivered is justified by specific circumstances and is formally declared by a state government, in recognition that crisis operations will be in effect for a sustained period. The formal declaration that crisis standards of care are in operation enables specific legal/regulatory powers and protections for healthcare providers in the necessary tasks of allocating and using scarce medical resources and implementing alternate care facility operations. (IOM 2009, 2)

To achieve a system of just care, the IOM (2009) devised the following vision for crisis standards of care:

- Fairness: All those affected by the standards should recognize them as fair.
- Equitable processes: Decisions and implementation of standards must be made equitably.
- Community and provider engagement, education, and communication: Active collaboration with the public and stakeholders is needed.
- The rule of law: Authorities can empower action and create an environment in which to implement the crisis standards through laws that support the standards and create appropriate incentives.

The Center for Biosecurity of the University of Pittsburgh Medical Center (UPMC 2010a) provides leadership guidance to top health officials and government leaders during crisis events, such as bioterrorism or epidemics—events that are embroiled with immense political and social pressure for decisive and visible action. They state, "the most common dilemmas facing past leaders have been balancing disease control imperatives with those of individual liberty, economic stability, and preventing stigma."

Comprehensive Exercise Program

Plans are just one step in the coordination of disaster response and relief delivery. Understanding and implementing effective plans requires

- individuals trained on the tasks they must perform,
- groups trained in their collective tasks, and
- leaders who are empowered to make independent, situation-based decisions.

The organization's preparedness is incomplete unless the EOP is tied to a comprehensive exercise and evaluation program. A comprehensive exercise program starts with appropriate drills and leads to progressively complex exercises, until the exercises are as close to reality as possible.

To ensure an efficient and effective response, training must be addressed at three levels:

1. Individual
2. Collective (complex, team-oriented emergency management tasks)
3. Leader development (to develop and strengthen response professionalism, skills, and knowledge)

BUSINESS CRISIS AND CONTINUITY PLANNING

Crisis Management

Crisis situations are novel and unstructured. They lie outside of our typical operating framework. They are highly uncertain and complex situations that require nonprogrammed responses and are characterized by an overload of incomplete and conflicting information. The process of perceiving, selecting, and processing this information is critical to effective crisis management (Reilly 1993).

Crisis characteristics include (Post 1993):

- Threats to major values
- Time urgency

- Ambiguity or uncertainty
- Surprise or uniqueness

Disasters affect everyone—customers, supply chain, insurers—and could permanently alter a business and community. *Two out of five companies that experience a disaster will go out of business within five years* (Gartner, Inc. 2001). This statistic leaves little room for healthcare leaders to ignore the need to prepare their organizations at every level.

> A fundamental mission for crisis managers is to prevent loss of control before a crisis happens, prevent further loss of control when a crisis arises, and when and where possible regain control when loss of control happens. Regaining control of a crisis situation becomes a central principle of crisis management. (Heath 1997)

Healthcare organizations exist to provide products, care, and services to the community and patients who seek them, and even in the most critical situations they must strive to maintain or restore their capability to do so. Many businesses can choose to shut down during a crisis, but not hospitals (Shaw 2006).

Business crisis and continuity management refers to "the business management practices that provide the focus and guidance for the decisions and actions necessary for a business to prevent, prepare for, respond to, recover, restore and transition from a disruptive (crisis) event in a manner consistent with its strategic objectives" (Shaw and Harrald 2004, 3). Organizational functions—such as risk management, contingency planning, crisis management, emergency response, and business resumption and recovery—are established based on the organization's perception of its environment and risks.

Shaw (2006) also noted from the work of Ian Mitroff (2001) that most businesses do not have an adequate crisis management program, supported by corporate culture, individual- and organizational-level expertise, infrastructure, and plans and procedures to fully understand, prepare for, and manage the crises they may face. He further stated that the vast majority of organizations and institutions have not been designed to anticipate crises or to manage them effectively once they have occurred. Neither the mechanics nor the basic skills are in place for effective crisis management (Mitroff 2001).

Corporate-Level Crisis Management

A large organization or multifacility system should have a headquarters emergency operations center (EOC) and fully integrated facility plans that reflect the role of corporate support and resources that may be employed in a crisis situation. The following should be considered when planning the EOC:

- Location
  - Avoid high-risk areas.
  - Consider potential natural events that could trigger technological events, such as power outages to the EOC.
  - Choose an area that is accessible to all and allow operating space for large numbers.
  - Choose an area that is safe and secure, 24/7.
- Structure/Infrastructure.
  - Make sure it is appropriate for the risk profile of the area.
    - Self-sufficient
    - Includes back-up utilities
    - Has alternate communication systems
    - Personnel health and sanitation are covered
  - Include adequate and appropriate space and furniture for catastrophic-level work.
  - Include appropriate supplies and equipment for an efficient EOC operation.
  - Preselect alternate sites for operation centers, if needed.

Resilience

Effective enterprise-wide IT and infrastructure risk and business resilience planning should be at the heart of your business. Maintaining operational stability can affect revenue and even long-term survival (IBM 2010).

Resilience is the ability to adjust to expected or unexpected stress and to restore equilibrium when confronted with trauma, tragedy, and threat (Steinberg and Ritzmann 1990). At the community level, it is the capacity for social units (individuals, communities, people, and groups) to lessen the negative effects of hazards and to implement recovery activities to limit social disruption and the effects on future events.

Enhancing community resilience can strengthen preparedness and prevent or reduce adverse consequences associated with disasters. The same is true for business resilience. Aquirre (2006) states that "resilience is both the capacity of a system to react appropriately to moments of crises that have not been entirely anticipated, and its ability to anticipate these crises and to enact, through planning and recovery, changes in the systems that will mitigate their effects. It is a never-ending open process, for the sources of often unanticipated demands that create changes in the known dynamics of the system are multiple."

The four properties of resilience identified by Bruneau and colleagues (2003) are:

1. Robustness—strength to withstand the stress
2. Redundancy—substitutable elements, systems, and responses
3. Resourcefulness—the ability to identify problems, formulate priorities, and creatively apply resources to accomplish the organization's goals
4. Rapidity—the ability to address, prioritize, and accomplish goals in a timely manner so as to contain losses and prevent future disruption

All four are critical components of a solid healthcare facility plan for responding to catastrophic events. "Building a disaster resilient business will reduce costs, limit exposures, and maintain operational continuity while protecting employees, property, reputation, corporate value, and competitive marketplace position" (IBM 2010).

The Key Elements of Building Business Resiliency Within Public and Private Sectors
Brent H. Woodworth, CEO of LA Preparedness Foundation and founder and past head of IBM's Crisis Response Team, provided this response when asked "What are the key elements of building business resiliency within public and private sectors?"

Well, there are quite a few, and let me at least get the top five to be considered by your audience...

1. One of the first is looking at issues such as communication and information management. Those two elements are key cornerstones of any plan put together. Communications: if you can't call for help, you can't get help. You really must be able to communicate. And on information, the information required to make critical decisions in a disaster, is frankly, just as important as food, water, or shelter in a crisis; because if you can't get the right information to meet the needs of the victims, you can't supply them with what they require. So, those two elements become the first component I would address.

2. The second one is to break down the stovepipes or silos to communication among organizations. While having organizations that are measured in a concise manner from a work or government standpoint may make sense in our daily lives, when a disaster hits, it doesn't work because Mother Nature closes every single one of those silos and comes back and says "if you don't share information effectively across your departments, you can't respond in an effective manner." So, we need to break through those silos by communicating properly.

3. Another issue [is] the emergency powers provisions. A lot of government agencies and businesses have certain policies and practices in place for normal daily

---

business. In a disaster, we need to find ways to not just "bend the rules" but put in place alternative rules or "emergency powers" that apply to help the victims of a disaster much more effectively. Those may be changes in customs regulations, or change in a tax that can be deferred for some reason. It may be making it easier to get building permits at zero cost and automating the process. But each of those would come under a category called "emergency powers provisions."

4. The next is developing "task orders" in advance. What is a task order? A task order is something for a business or government entity, again, that defines a particular procedure or process that is needed to respond in a disaster. It may be procuring a certain item. It may be buying telephones or services, or computers or procuring pencils—whatever it is, but in the normal routine they go through a long cycle to get these things approved. In a disaster, you don't have that kind of time. So if you can define those elements in advance and go through your approval processes ahead of time and create these task orders, when a disaster occurs, it is then very easy to issue those at the time of the event and get a response immediately instead of waiting the two, three or four days or sometimes weeks to accomplish what you need.

5. The last item is a non-binding memorandum of understanding (MOU). Now, an MOU is a document that's signed between two parties that allows them to more effectively share information in a crisis. This can be between the public and the private sector, or within the public sector it can be across multiple agencies.

Remember I mentioned disasters breaking down stovepipes and silos? Well, the MOU helps to document that process—and, for example, after the tragic events of Hurricane Katrina, one of the challenges was trying to reunify families and get them together. Well, there were many agencies involved that had information that was key—the Red Cross, who was in the shelters, the hospitals, the morgue—many other agencies that were involved. If an MOU to share that information had been signed in advance across these agencies, then the reunification process could potentially be accelerated and each component could do due diligence in advance. Then, when the disaster occurred we would be more effective in responding to the needs of the victims.

Another great example is public and private sector partnerships. If the private sector provided a non-binding MOU where they were talking about the kinds of services and support that they might be able to provide at no cost in a disaster (donations of food or services or materials or in-kind capabilities) and that was collected in a database that was available to the public sector to help manage in a disaster, then the public and private sectors could work together in a crisis and accelerate the delivery of critical services to the point of the victims in a faster, more efficient manner. So, I'm a big fan of these MOUs and how that would work.

(continued)

RISK MANAGEMENT

Sociologist Niklas Luhmann is credited with this popular definition of *risk*: "the threat or probability that an action or event will adversely or beneficially affect an organization's ability to achieve its objectives." It is, more simply, the uncertainty of an outcome.

Qualitatively, risk is proportional to the losses that may result from an event and the probability that the event will occur. Greater loss and greater event likelihood equals greater overall risk:

$$Risk = [Probability\ of\ an\ event\ occurring] \times [Impact\ of\ the\ event]$$

Risk management is the foundation of a comprehensive business continuity and contingency management (BCCM) program and drives all decisions that affect other functions in the framework. It is a continual and iterative process that requires dialogue with multiple stakeholders and monitoring and adjustment in light of changes to the environment.

The protection of personnel, property, and reputation and the ability to recover, resume, and restore business operations according to a reasoned and defendable plan are inherent in an organization's planning and preparedness. The business area analysis and business impact analysis provide an economic basis for risk-based decision making and the allocation of resources supporting the overall risk management function (Shaw 2006).

The risk certain events pose to your operation should be examined in light of the probability that the event will occur (high to low) and the effect the event may have on your continuity of operations (high to low). Exhibit 3.1 illustrates examples of various disasters and where they may fall in your personalized risk matrix. For example, the probability of an earthquake may be low, but the effect on healthcare operations would be high. Flooding is the most frequently experienced disaster; thus, the probability of a flood is high. Whether rising water impacts the community or the healthcare facility itself, the resulting effect on healthcare operations would most likely be high.

Exhibit 3.1 Disaster Risk Matrix

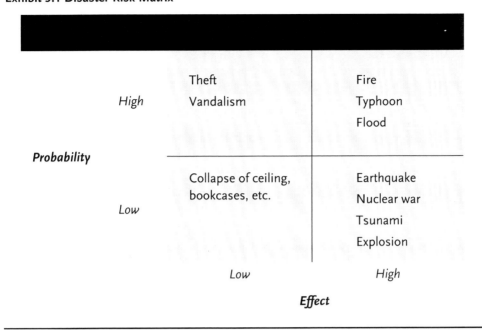

		Low	High
Probability	High	Theft Vandalism	Fire Typhoon Flood
	Low	Collapse of ceiling, bookcases, etc.	Earthquake Nuclear war Tsunami Explosion
		Low	High

Effect

Risk in Private Sector Healthcare

Since a majority of America's critical infrastructure is managed by the private sector, the "private sector generally remains the first line of defense for its own facilities" (Bullock and Haddow 2006, 257). Private sector healthcare facilities should "reassess and adjust their planning, assurance and investment programs to better accommodate the increased risk presented by deliberate actions of violence" (White House 2003). The primary federal planning documents (the NRF and NIMS) include the private sector in all phases of crisis and emergency awareness, prevention, preparedness, response and recovery planning, and operations, and the National Response Plan (DHS 2004) explicitly charges the private sector to enhance overall readiness.

NFPA 1600 Standard on Disaster/Emergency Management and Business Continuity Program

Though voluntary, the National Fire Protection Association's (2004) NFPA 1600 Standard on Disaster/Emergency Management and Business Continuity Program has been recognized as the national standard for private sector preparedness. The

9/11 Commission (2004) states that "private-sector preparedness is not a luxury; it is a cost of doing business in the post-9/11 world. It is ignored at a tremendous potential cost in lives, money, and national security." The NFPA 1600 defines a business continuity program as "an ongoing process supported by senior management and funded to ensure that the necessary steps are taken to identify the impact of potential losses, maintain viable recovery strategies and recovery plans, and ensure continuity of services through personnel training, plant testing, and maintenance."

The NFPA 1600 2004 edition Disaster/Emergency Management and Business Continuity Program specifies 15 program elements:

1. General
2. Law and authorities
3. Hazard identification, risk assessment, and impact analysis
4. Hazard mitigation
5. Resource management
6. Mutual aid
7. Planning
8. Direction, control, and coordination
9. Communications and warning
10. Operations and procedures
11. Logistics and facilities
12. Training
13. Exercises, evaluations, and corrective actions
14. Crisis communication and public information
15. Finance and administration

Shaw (2006) presents a framework hierarchy of the multiple functions that require integration and coordination for the sake of program effectiveness and efficiency. The framework divides activities into those that occur before a crisis, those that occur during the crisis event, and those that occur after the crisis. The components (top to bottom) and their phases in time are presented in Exhibit 3.2.

EXTERNAL FRAMEWORK

Healthcare facilities must plan as much for the external collaboration and integration required as for internal collaboration. This external framework includes

- community interoperability,
- creating an integrated and interoperable system (ICS and HICS),
- focusing on guidelines and agreements for mutual assistance and aid, and
- collaboration and building healthcare coalitions.

Exhibit 3.2 Crisis Functions

Hierarchy of Functions	Definition	Phase of Crisis Event
Enterprise management	The systematic understanding and management of business operations within the context of the organization's culture, beliefs, mission, objectives, and organizational structure	All
Crisis management	The coordination of efforts to control a crisis event consistent with the organization's strategic goals. Generally associated with response, recovery, and resumption operations during and following a crisis event, these responsibilities extend to pre-event mitigation, prevention, and preparedness, and post-event restoration and transition.	During
Crisis communication	All means of communication, internal and external to an organization, designed and delivered to support the crisis management function	Late event and after
Knowledge management (environmental monitoring, sensing, and detection; organizational learning)	The acquisition, assurance, representation, transformation, transfer, and use of information supporting enterprise management	All
Risk management (risk-based decision making, risk assessment, business area analysis, business impact analysis, risk communication)	The synthesis of the risk tools and decision-making functions to make strategic and tactical decisions on how business risks will be treated—whether they will be ignored, reduced, transferred, or avoided	Before
Planning	Based on the results of risk management and within the overall context of enterprise management, the development of plans, policies, and procedures to address the risks that are above the level of acceptance to a business, its assets, and its stakeholders Plans may stand alone or be consolidated, but they must be integrated.	Before
Program implementation	The implementation and management of specific programs (such as physical security, cyber security, environmental health, occupational health, safety, etc.) within the context of enterprise management	All

(continued)

Exhibit 3.2 (continued)

Hierarchy of Functions	Definition	Phase of Crisis Event
Systems monitoring	Measuring and evaluating program performance in the context of the enterprise as an overall system of interrelated parts	All
Awareness/training/ exercising	A tiered program to develop and maintain individual, team, and organizational awareness and preparedness, ranging from individual and group familiarization and skill-based training through full organizational exercises	Before
Incident management	The management of operations, logistics, planning, finance, administration, safety, and information flow associated with the operational response to the effects of a crisis event	All
Incident response	The tactical reaction to the effects of a crisis event to protect personnel and property, assess and stabilize the situation, and conduct response operations that support the economic viability of a business	All
Business continuity (business recovery, business resumption)	The business-specific plans and actions that enable an organization to respond to a crisis event in a manner such that business functions, subfunctions, and processes are recovered and resumed according to a predetermined plan, prioritized by their criticality to the economic viability of the business	During and after
Restoration and transition	Plans and actions to restore and transition a business to "new normal" operations following a crisis event	During and after

Source: Shaw (2006). Used with permission.

Community Interoperability

Catastrophic events have great interdependency, and their effects snowball. When one network fails, the impact is magnified. Information services are highly networked and tied into the availability of electrical power; both systems are vulnerable to disruptions that can take weeks or months to reset. Financial losses can be so high that no single source is able to cover them (Ruback, Wells, and Bissell 2009, 4).

Yet, healthcare executives rarely investigate the preparedness of public sector services for disaster or operation in catastrophic events. This oversight can leave a healthcare facility vulnerable. Healthcare leaders must meet with and be familiar with the leaders of all other community organizations. This "meet and greet" effort often leads to development of integrated plans that strengthen the response of all organizations to a catastrophic event.

Following and practicing ICS and HICS integrate all planning efforts and ensure that they are interoperable. This is critical to communication, which is consistently the number one area of concern in disaster response. Whether the weakness is incompatibility of communications equipment or a failure to communicate and exchange thoughts, plans, and actions, it can be addressed with effective planning and follow-through.

Creating an Integrated and Interoperable System: ICS and IMS

In 1970, two devastating wildfires burned over 600,000 acres of Southern California. As multiple jurisdictions were involved in the response, Firefighting Resources of Southern California Organized for Potential Emergencies (FIRESCOPE) received congressional funding to develop a coordinated response mechanism for incidents. The resulting ICS provided a standardized emergency incident management system (IMS), which has since also been adopted by hospitals (Auf der Heide 1996, 467).

The IMS is a systems approach to managing an emergency situation where more than one organization or entity is involved. IMS has become the nationally accepted standard for managing emergencies. This approach is organized by function. All services and personnel are arranged under the distinct functional areas of planning, operations, logistics, and finance. Most responder/clinical staff align under the operations function. All functional area leaders report to the incident commander.

The success of IMS lies in its key provisions of

- common terminology,
- integrated communications,
- modular organization,
- a unified management structure,
- a manageable span of control,
- consolidated action plans, and
- comprehensive resource management.

IMS/ICS has expanded to the healthcare facility setting, where HICS and similar models are now used. All hospitals should have implemented HICS or some form of IMS that conforms to that practiced throughout the community (Boatright and McGlown 2005).

The primary functions of the HICS are listed in Exhibit 3.3.

Guidelines/Agreements for Mutual Aid and Assistance

Healthcare institutions benefit from preexisting agreements to provide services and resources or to assist others in their need for the same. Memoranda of understanding

Exhibit 3.3 Primary Functions of HICS

HICS Functional Areas	Responsibilities
Command	The Incident Commander: • Provides frontline leadership and management; in command • Provides tactical planning and execution • Communicates needs to the city/county or state EOC • Could be predesignated (private sector) or the first senior official on the scene (public sector) • Has capability and authority to assume control • Assesses the situation • Implements the EM plan • Determines appropriate response strategies • Activates resources • Oversees all response activities • Expands resources or ICS structure as the event escalates • Declares the end of the event • Leads post-event follow-up
Planning	Gathering, evaluating, and disseminating information about the event and status of resources
Operations	Managing all tactical operations
Logistics	Providing the supplies, services, and facilities to support the incident
Finance/ Administration	Providing financial oversight and direction, including cost recovery, contracts, and personnel administrative services

(MOU) or agreement (MOA) and mutual aid agreements (MAAs) are nonbinding but must be addressed well in advance of need. You can't negotiate in the middle of a disaster. Relying on assistance from other providers or agreeing to assist in their need is an exercise in trust building and relationship strengthening.

A hospital or healthcare organization should identify all stakeholders and service providers on whom it may rely for assistance in disasters. Using the HVA, the hospital can prioritize these stakeholders and services by the greatest likelihood of need. The agreement must be in writing, and MOUs and MOAs should be reviewed at least annually and after each event or pre-established period of critique or assessment (an exercise in which agreements are activated). Keep these documents current and the relationships behind them strong.

Collaboration and Building Healthcare Coalitions

The UPMC identified community-based collaboration among institutions and agencies in the healthcare sector as essential to preparedness for mass casualty events. *The Medical Surge Capacity and Capability (MSCC) Handbook*, the Joint Commission standards, and the Hospital Preparedness Program (HPP) guidance all emphasize the importance of such cooperation. Without it, healthcare institutions would be unable to respond optimally to large mass casualty events—and certainly catastrophic-level health events—through ICS and HICS.

The latest collaborative push is toward the development of healthcare coalitions. Though designs vary, the UPMC (2010b) defined this as "a formal collaboration among hospitals, public health, and EMAs that may include other nonhospital healthcare entities. …Fully functional and mature healthcare coalitions have a role in preparedness and response."

Healthcare coalitions have emerged and are in various stages of development. Much of the U.S. healthcare system is still not represented. Many coalitions are not yet fully declared or functional in preparedness and response. A great need remains to fund and guide the development of coalitions around the country using a common, yet flexible, set of functional criteria.

Appendix 3.1: What CEOs Need to Know About Training and Exercises

1. You only respond as well as you practice. Response training and exercises increase your ability to appropriately react when a disaster strikes.
2. Emergency preparedness isn't all that different from golf, tennis, or your kid's piano lessons—practice makes perfect. Your facility has an emergency response plan, but if you don't practice it, you won't be able to respond appropriately.
3. Having a plan, practicing the plan, and having confidence in your organization to effectively implement the plan will allow you to quickly move from disaster mode to normal operations.
4. Consider designating a small group of clinical directors or other upper-level managers as your incident commanders. Your administrative team can then support this group for drills and real incidents.
5. It is important for you and the rest of the administrative team to develop an awareness of emergency preparedness so you know what is happening in your facility and to support your incident management team.
6. Training is vital to keep your staff up to date and engaged in emergency preparedness. Just as continuing medical education keeps clinical skills sharp and makes an employee more valuable, so does training on emergency preparedness. When finances are a concern there are great free training courses available through FEMA and other organizations.
7. By encouraging each shift to talk though their potential response to an event during their watch, they get in the habit of preidentifying patients who could be discharged and how to manage an emergency situation. This makes the appropriate response second nature.
8. Training and exercises are required in the Joint Commission accreditation process, as well as for National Incident Management System compliance.
9. Exercises are an excellent way to connect with the community and garner positive media coverage. You are actively demonstrating your commitment to excellence in all areas.
10. You need to set the tone and expectations for exercise and training. Make

it a part of job responsibilities and a part of annual evaluations. In this way, employees won't feel as though they are not doing their "real" jobs when participating in training or exercises.

Source:
Melinda Johnson, MPP
MMRS Program Coordinator
Denver Metropolitan Medical Response System
Denver Health & Hospital Authority, Denver, CO
October 2009

Appendix 3.2: Preparing for a Crisis

1. Clearly define what is most important to your organization and communicate that to every member of your organization and to your stakeholders. Knowing what is most important can help guide decisions and actions during disruptive events.
2. Based upon what is important and how you envision the future of your organization, develop a comprehensive and realistic strategy that includes protecting your organization before, during, and after a disruptive event. Remember, hope is not a strategy.
3. Remember that you are in business and that an overarching goal is to remain in business during and after a disruptive event. Actions taken in the exigency of the moment should not threaten your continuity of operations in the long term.
4. Invest in preparing for disruptive events, but do not stop at just planning. Moving from preparedness to real readiness involves a continuous cycle of training, testing, exercising, and maintaining plans at all levels of the organization.
5. Engage your local authorities (police, fire, emergency medical services, and emergency management) in your preparedness efforts. They are both a resource and a partner in your efforts.
6. Encourage (or even require) every member of your organization to develop and maintain a personal/family preparedness plan and have organizational leaders set the example with their own plans.
7. Inform your preparedness resourcing decisions with a sound risk management process. Realize that risk information is often fraught with uncertainties and assumptions that must be questioned and considered when making decisions.
8. Define your crisis management organization, responsibilities, and protocols, and practice, practice, practice.
9. Develop and perfect crisis communication policies and procedures for both internal and external audiences.

10. Be involved in the efforts to protect your organization. Set the example for all to follow.

Source:
Gregory L. Shaw, DSc, CBCP
Associate Professor of Engineering Management; Co-director, Institute for Crisis, Disaster and Risk Management
George Washington University, Washington, DC
September 2009

Part II

RESPONSE

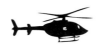

CHAPTER 4

Responding: You Are in This Alone

Phil Robinson

LEADERSHIP DURING A CRISIS

The most important leadership skill in any crisis is the ability to stay calm, focused, and confident. More than at any other time, the organization will reflect the personality and behavior of the leader during a critical challenge. The CEO is the face of the organization, and communication with all the people affected by the disaster—from your staff to patients to the media to emergency responders—is crucial.

Think back on the leaders who have impressed you at times of crisis and those who have not. Most likely, the former group displayed a hands-on, "roll up your sleeves" involvement. This is exactly what a leader should do in the heat of battle. And most important, a leader should assume nothing and leave nothing to chance.

- Don't assume that your message is delivered unless you deliver it yourself, via email or memo or in person.
- Don't assume that others know what is expected of them unless you clearly articulate those expectations well in advance of any sort of disaster.
- Don't assume that any other agency or organization is going to put your needs and the needs of those for whom you are responsible ahead of any others.

Only you will make sure that you get what you need when you need it.

Effective Leaders

The most effective leaders in a crisis

- are visible, practicing management by walking around (MBWA);
- are calm and focused;
- are rested (yes, you have to be well rested to be effective);
- assume nothing and leave nothing to chance;
- communicate constantly, internally and externally, remaining receptive to new information;
- manage the message and the media;
- have a plan and know how to execute it;
- realize that they may be unable to rely on outside help for at least three to four days;
- have prepared their organizations to be self-sufficient;
- are prepared to deal with the personal challenges and needs of the staff and their families;
- are not afraid to challenge the authority of the governmental and political infrastructure, whose flaws and dysfunctions will be exposed during this kind of event;
- define the primary elements of the situation;
- identify and consider the major values, interests, and objectives to be fulfilled and prioritize them based on the information at hand at that moment;
- search for and evaluate alternative courses of action;
- estimate probable costs and risks of alternatives;
- discriminate between relevant and irrelevant information;
- consider problems that arise in implementing options;
- assess the situation from the perspective of other parties;
- resist defensive procrastination and premature closure;
- monitor feedback from the developing situation; and
- make adjustments to meet real changes in the environment.

THE POLITICS OF DISASTER RESPONSE

A number of the healthcare CEOs and national leaders interviewed for this book confirmed that you are truly on your own in a major event. Depend only on yourself and your internal team. The lack of government help and the confusing and conflicting directions from local, state, and federal government agencies surprised many of our leaders.

Agencies at all levels must collaborate vertically and horizontally to prepare for an event. To ensure collaboration, the following factors must be addressed (Pine 2009).

- Disasters are political in nature and involve interorganizational conflict and blame.
- Conflict between organizations is part of response operations. Disagreements may evolve concerning some of the following issues:
  - Who will be given authority over incident command?
  - Which organizations will be assigned seemingly menial or less visible tasks?
  - Which organizations will be given additional resources and responsibilities?
  - Who will get credit or blame for the outcome of the event?
- Some organizations restrict communication and coordination with others simply because interorganizational rivalries exist.
  - Politics are prevalent when disasters are declared and when resources begin to be distributed. There may be disagreement about who should get help first, or major supporters may be favored, or those with significantly less power may be ignored.

Where's the Cavalry?
"FEMA was not helpful. They promised items would be delivered that never came." And when asked what you wish you had known before this event, the reply was "that promises made by FEMA should not be relied upon solely" (Dr. Thomas Royer, CEO of CHRISTUS Health. Excerpt from interview 2009).

Ward Off Conflict
Strategies to reduce interorganizational conflict in preparing for a catastrophe include the following (Pine 2009).

- Get to know the city leaders and the leaders of other organizations. Develop a rapport with them and encourage them to get to know each other.
- Plan together and clarify responsibilities before disaster strikes.
- Find consensus during preparations rather than resolve disagreements after response operations have begun.
- Show other organizations the merit of cooperation, communication, and coordination.
- Ask political figures for assistance.
- If all else fails, ask the mayor or county commissioner to settle differences or enforce decisions.

DECISION MAKING AND TOUGH ISSUES

Decision making is difficult in a catastrophe and during disaster response operations. Dror (1988) identifies the reasons.

- Disasters are characterized by injury, death, and destruction and demand the immediate attention of decision makers.
- Time is critical because lives and well-being are at stake.
- There is incredible pressure for decision makers to act quickly and even prematurely.
- There are no easy decisions.
- Uncertainty is an expected correlate of disasters.
- The physical and emotional demands placed on decision makers may impair effective decision making.

Most healthcare leaders activate their hospital command centers and work through and with their management team (the command staff under activation) to receive information and make decisions.

Decision-making processes rarely follow a set pattern. Instead, the pattern may become evident as the event unfolds and may include one or more of the following factors (Fink 1986):

- Vigilance: The leader follows a methodical, high-quality process to objectively collect available information, thoroughly consider it, search for other possible options, and make a well-reasoned decision.
- Unconflicted adherence: The leader continues with the current situation.
- Unconflicted change: The leader follows the last advice he or she received.
- Defensive avoidance: The leader avoids making decisions.
- Hypervigilance: The leader's approach vacillates.

Another pitfall the decision group may face is "groupthink" (Neck and Manz 1994). Groupthink refers to a mode of thinking in which people engage when they are deeply involved in a cohesive group. Members' striving for unanimity overrides their motivation to realistically appraise alternate courses of action. This results in a deterioration of mental efficiency, reality testing, and moral judgment. Groupthink can occur if the group is insulated, if the group leader has a preference for a certain decision, if the group lacks norms requiring methodical procedures, or if group members are homogeneous in social background and ideology. It may also occur as a result of high stress from external threat with low hope of a better solution than the leader's and low group self-esteem induced by the group's perception of recent failures, the excessive difficulty of current decision-making tasks, and moral dilemmas.

Neck and Manz (1994) state that the strategy to counter groupthink is to move toward "teamthink." This positive approach takes advantage of open discussion and team mental imagery to create a common vision. Teamthink can occur in a group that encourages divergent views and open expression of concerns and ideas, is aware of limitations and threats, recognizes each member's uniqueness, and discusses its collective doubts.

Even in the best decision-making environment, a healthcare leader may make critical mistakes in the decision process. Crisis-induced stress, whether it results from a perceived threat to one's values or simply from anxiety or fear, alters the leader's coping pattern. This affects information processing and decision choice. And as stress increases, performance often decreases.

Post (1993) lists symptoms of defective decision making in a crisis:

- Giving major attention to the immediate consequences of an action and diminished attention to its long-range consequences
- Perceived requirement for decisional closure, which may lead to premature action
- In searching for certainty, a tendency toward irrational procrastination
- Cognitive rigidity—a tendency to maintain a fixed mind-set and not be open to new information

- A tendency to reduce cognitive complexity and uncertainty
- A tendency to reduce the range of options considered
- A tendency to "bolster"—to upgrade factors in favor of the preferred action and downgrade other factors
- Viewing the present in terms of the past
- A tendency to seek familiar patterns or to relate the critical events to mental schemata or scripts
- Diminished creativity
- A tendency toward the fundamental attribution bias—to see the others' actions as precipitated by internal causes rather than external circumstances
- A tendency to fall into the actor–observer discrepancy—to see the external situation as the cause of one's own behavior without attending to one's internal psychological motivations

Neck and Manz (1994) would add to this list:

- Incomplete survey of alternatives
- Incomplete survey of objectives
- Failure to examine the risks of preferred choices
- Failure to reappraise initially rejected alternatives
- Poor information search
- Selective bias in processing information at hand
- Failure to work out contingency plans

Post (1993) describes three common personalities and how they perform under crisis-induced stress. The *compulsive leader* often becomes paralyzed by indecision and tends toward irrational procrastination for fear of making a mistake. Once this type of leader makes a decision, it is difficult to reopen it. A compulsive leader is most comfortable applying set policies and procedures to solve problems. He or she is sensitive to the leadership hierarchy, is overly responsive to superiors, competes with peers, and dominates subordinates.

The *narcissistic personality* is self-centered, egocentric, and self-absorbed. A leader who fits this profile seeks constant reassurance of his self-worth. The narcissistic leader's primary loyalty is to himself, so he acts to promote his own position and can shift positions easily. Narcissists believe that they are principled and scrupulous individuals. They seek advisors who prop up their self-esteem.

The *paranoid personality* feels surrounded by enemies and is extremely suspicious of the motivations of others. A paranoid leader has difficulty trusting his or her subordinates. This type of leader reaches conclusions before gathering evidence to support them, then seeks evidence to support those conclusions.

Dror (1988) also lists some strategies for effective decision making during disaster response.

- Design preferable models. Study the situation or problem in detail, determining the gap that exists between the goal and reality and intervening to adapt the process to the desired outcome.
- Debug. Observe the decision process to correct potential weaknesses and mistakes as they become apparent.
- Think critically. People often fail to think outside the box.

Leadership Wisdom During Crisis

"The surest sign of a crisis is that when you have a major problem, no one tries to tell you how to do your job. Small problems produce a plethora of ideas and suggestions on what you should be doing, which are strangely absent when a big problem hits" (Gilbert 1982).

The following suggestions are guidelines for managing during a crisis (Gilbert 1982).
- Don't make it worse.
- Capture control of the information flow. The problem is usually too much information, not too little. Establish reliable filters to help isolate you from all the input clamoring for your attention. Others need an overview of what you are doing to provide support.
- Save yourself for the main events. You can't possibly do everything, so put problems in "boxes" and delegate early. The ad hoc crisis management environment is a special form of delegation, and some time must be spent defining the boxes and what is to be done with them.
- Refuse to be drawn into trivial matters. Demands will be made that you personally deal with even the most mundane problems. Don't do it. Keep your focus on important matters and positively refuse to deal with anything else. At times, dealing with little problems can be satisfying, because we can't come to grips with the big ones. Avoiding trivia requires discipline.
- Insist helpers get adequate rest. This rule applies to you as well, and if you don't follow it, no one else will. You should start assigning enforced rest periods to your people almost immediately. Silly people will continue to be silly. People will act irrationally; rivalries will surface. Crisis situations tend to bring out the best and worst in all of us. It is our responsibility as managers to understand people, make use of their strengths, and mitigate their weaknesses.
- Make sure everyone knows what's happening. Bring key organizations and people together often to disseminate and exchange views. People and organizations react

(continued)

irrationally when they perceive a dearth of information. Voids are filled with rumors and speculation. Insist on economy of communication. People can communicate succinctly if they try.

- Select a good boss.
- Return to normal operations ASAP.
- Litigation may follow. Keep a good audit trail of reports, actions, conditions, and decisions to facilitate your defense, should it be necessary.
- Beware of abdicators. Do not let individuals or organizations abdicate their responsibilities. You may need them. Hold their feet to the fire and insist they carry out their responsibilities regardless of how painful it may be to them.
- Know your territory. Know other organizations' capabilities, limitations, and lines of communication well in advance. A time of crisis is not the time to get to know people.
- Critically reexamine assumptions. Here and in everyday arrangements, most of our decisions are based on assumptions. Critical reviews and updates of all assumptions going into the decision-making process are vital.
- Feed the media. They will go through three phases: (1) stunned by tragedy, (2) accusation (early after the initial shock, the hunt for someone to blame begins), and (3) the story behind the news, or the search for controversy. (What really happened and why?)
- Provide for survivor needs. Survivors have an overwhelming need for reassurance that they are alive. This will be expressed in the need to touch others and be touched, to talk out their feelings, and to be reunited with their loved ones.
- Do what you should do. Have the courage to do what you know is best. We must have the courage to do what is right regardless of the consequences, not only for successful management of the crisis, but for our own peace of mind. We cannot live comfortably with failure to do what we knew was right at the time.

CHALLENGES DURING A CRISIS

Healthcare leaders face a number of difficult challenges in large-scale events. The sections that follow cover the most commonly discussed challenges.

Evacuation or Influx of Patients

One of the biggest challenges is preparing for an influx of patients and the need to quickly evacuate the entire facility. Huge shifts in volume need to be planned for well in advance. The need to move large numbers of people into or out of your facility requires tremendous coordination with other organizations and agencies that may not follow through on their commitments.

Having adequate staff and supplies to get you through at least the first three or four days of the disaster means having food, water, fuel, bedding, supplies, drugs, power, and more to meet every need of the staff and their families, the doctors and their families, the patients and their families, and all the others who hunker down in your hospital. This places a great burden on the entire infrastructure, especially the supply chain and support staff, and requires you to provide services you may not normally have to (e.g., pet care, child care, accommodations for entire families).

Staffing the Facility During a Disaster

As mentioned earlier in this chapter, setting the expectations for the staff well before an event occurs is essential. I have the staff in my hospital read and sign the disaster response policy, which states their obligations to be at work in the event of a storm or other catastrophe, at the beginning of each hurricane season. Even higher standards are set for the leadership team.

Of course, you can hardly ask your associates to leave their families—including their pets—behind in the event of an approaching storm, so the organization has an obligation to provide shelter and support for their two- and four-legged loved ones for the duration. Your emergency staffing should ensure that you have enough people to staff your facility for many days, while allowing the employees adequate breaks and rest time between shifts. In catastrophic events, it may be days or weeks before the relief staff can make it into the hospital, so make sure you have enough core staff to run the facility and take care of your patients until well after the crisis is over.

It is strongly suggested that you ask every individual you are sheltering to sign a set of "rules of conduct" that clearly defines what is expected of them as guests in your facility.

Staff Willingness to Report to Work

Qureshi and colleagues (2005), among others, have conducted extensive research into healthcare workers' (HCWs) ability and willingness to report to duty during catastrophic disasters. Their findings addressed HCWs' *ability* and *willingness* to report (or not) for duty, as shown in Exhibit 4.1.

Exhibit 4.1 Healthcare Workers' Willingness to Report

HCWs were most able to report to work in a(n)

- Mass casualty incident (MCI) (83%)
- Environmental disaster (81%)
- Chemical event (71%)

And least able to report during a

- Smallpox epidemic (69%)
- Radiological event (64%)
- Sudden acute respiratory distress syndrome (SARS) outbreak (64%)
- Severe snowstorm (49%)

HCWs were most willing to report to work during a(n)

- Snowstorm (80%)
- MCI (86%)
- Environmental disaster (84%)

And least willing to report during a

- SARS outbreak (48%)
- Radiological event (57%)
- Smallpox epidemic (61%)
- Chemical event (68%)

Source: Data from Qureshi et al. (2005).

Current evidence indicates that factors related to this willingness (or lack of it) include (Chaffee 2009)

- the type of disaster,
- concern for family, and
- concerns about personal safety.

Barriers to willingness to work include

- pet care needs and
- lack of personal protective equipment.

Medical Staff Issues

It can be difficult to get or keep medical staff on site during a disaster response. Many physicians are members of the medical staffs of multiple facilities. Do you know with which facility their loyalty lies?

You need the medical staff leadership on site to deal with uncovered medical services, disrupted call teams, physicians who failed to sign out their patients, and other issues. Medical staff officers should deal with physician issues during the crisis, and the best practice is to set up a medical command center adjacent to your incident command center.

Disasters can give rise to some unique medical staff issues.

- Physicians are unable to come to the hospital to care for their patients.
- Some critical medical services are covered inadequately or not at all.
- Physicians and their families may be unwilling to follow the rules of the facility and become major distractions during the response efforts.
- The hospital-based departments are especially integral in management and treatment of injuries, especially the emergency department, radiology, and anesthesia, so you may need specific disaster policies and plans to ensure that these are covered.
- House staff, if available, can fill gaps in the medical staff for the duration of the disaster and response to it.
- Triage and assessment needs may be great, especially if you have many patients, injuries, or casualties. You may need to deploy all available medical staff to accomplish these tasks. It's best to have a physician leader make these key decisions, if possible. Set up a parallel medical staff command center to allow the physicians to manage the medical aspects of the response.

Security Issues

As the severity of a disaster increases, community members, your staff and employees, and their families may seek refuge in your facility. Whether you accept individuals for shelter under an existing policy or—worst-case scenario—you experience a completely unplanned and unanticipated influx of individuals, the safety and security of your patients, your staff and employees, their families, and guests in your facility are paramount. This can be one of your greatest challenges. Under extreme conditions, you may need to control access to your facility or even create a lockdown situation to gain and maintain control in times of chaos.

Controlled access means limiting access to the facility to one or more entrances and exits, each manned by security personnel or by individuals with special training for this role. Those approved to enter or exit the facility will be preidentified on a list or by a visible means of security clearance (e.g., must show a photo ID badge, wear a facility-issued armband). Lockdown is a complete restriction of entrance into or exit from you facility. Extra security staff and a lockdown plan are essential to managing a crisis. Managing who comes into and leaves your facility protects your patients, your staff, and the physical plant, so there's no such thing as overkill in this area. Even when they leave no victims, storms and other disasters cause all kinds of people to descend on hospitals, so you must carefully manage and limit access points. If there are victims who require treatment, managing your intake and triage process is not only critical, it is a requirement of your disaster plan.

The Media

The media presents an additional challenge that the added security will help you manage, especially when it comes to protecting patient privacy and confidentiality. Disasters generate tremendous media interest, and most representatives of the press aren't the least bit concerned about HIPAA, infection control, privacy, or your image.

Gilbert (1982) suggests the following guidelines for dealing with the media.

- Establish fair and uniform rules. These will be followed scrupulously if you enforce them.
- Never put yourself in an adversarial position, regardless of the provocation.
- Establish good access for your media spokesperson and ensure that she remains fully informed so that she maintains credibility.
- Don't let questioners put words into your mouth.
- Be the media's conscience if necessary. Don't let them force the situation out of control.

Supply and Resupply

This is another area where it is difficult to overplan. It is too late to stock up on emergency supplies when your area is being evacuated before a storm or you are dealing with the aftermath of an earthquake. Depending on how many days of emergency supplies and food you have on hand prior to the disaster, resupply can become a bigger challenge than the initial purchase of emergency stock.

The entire greater Houston area was without fuel, ice, and other essentials for many days after Hurricane Ike in 2008. And after Hurricane Katrina in 2005, the only way to get essential supplies to the hospitals in New Orleans that had survived the storm was via helicopter. Part of your disaster planning has to be determining the levels of emergency supplies you need on hand at any given time. If you get advance warning of a pending event, as in a hurricane or winter storm, you need to determine what other supplies you should add to your stockpile.

WORKING THE PLAN

Your emergency operations plan, or EOP, should be a living, breathing document that is modified routinely to reflect changes in laws, regulations, recent disaster experiences, and changes in your organization and facility. The EOP is the framework that will guide you and your team through the response to the disaster. In addition to following the plan, here are some tips for effectively managing the plan and improving it each time you use it.

- Document everything you do—every decision, every delegation, every call you make, and every instruction you give or receive.
- Appoint a scribe to document all activity in the command center. This will pay great dividends after the dust has settled, and it certainly enhances your reimbursement documentation.
- Make clear handoffs of the leadership of the crisis management, even when you leave the room for just a few minutes. An effective change of command for the hospital command center should be practiced in every drill or exercise.
- Put as many of your directions in writing as possible, using email and your website if you can. If you do not use memos, newsletters or recorded messages are equally effective. Otherwise, you will be dealing with an exaggerated version of the child's game Telephone, where the message may be mangled beyond recognition by the time it reaches its intended audience, and it may not provide the leadership direction your staff needs.
- Maintain order in the command center. This is a serious operation, and the activities and problems being addressed may be cumulative and stressful. Provide a restful environment, but do not let it become a social hub or entertainment center for the facility leadership. A certain amount of levity is useful in extremely stressful situations, and humor (especially dark humor) may relieve stress. Monitor the mood and tension levels of your command staff, and ensure that their needs and the needs of other hospital employees and staff are met.
- Conduct your after-action review (AAR) or hot wash immediately. Even if you are exhausted, take time to evaluate your plan, determine what worked and what didn't, and change it as necessary. You may conduct this

after-action process at regular intervals throughout an extended exercise or event, but a global evaluative process must be completed at the termination of the event. In an extended disaster, staff may be tired and may need to collect their thoughts before conducting a leadership-wide AAR. However, encourage staff to write notes that address the critical elements of the AAR, and do not wait so long that the collective memory of the difficult issues is lost.

- The critical elements of an effective after-action report include the answers to the following questions.
    - What went well?
    - What opportunities for improvement exist?
    - What quick fixes can we make for the next time period or the long-term future?

A Pocket Primer for the Executive: Ten Steps in Disaster Planning
By Don Smithburg

Lesson 1(a)—Prepare for Disaster
Know your disaster plan no matter what your position is in the organization. Leaders better know it well, or have someone close by who is fluent and can help advise the leader. All of management should know how the plan works and where its deficits lay. If you operate multiple facilities, make sure field leaders know their respective roles in a disaster. Reviewing the emergency preparedness plan annually takes one or two hours at most. Refreshing the plan should be a perpetual process, just as updating the organization's strategic plan should be ingrained into the corporate culture.

Lesson 1(b)—Especially for Hospitals
Hospital emergency preparedness plans, if properly devised, should guide the response to any foreseeable disasters. A hospital that operates a major trauma center should be prepared to help other area hospitals, too. If the hospital is the only healthcare facility, or one of a few in a community, prepare for mass casualties as if it is a trauma center. A hospital association or similar consortium typically has communitywide disaster planning as a key duty, and also should liaison with FEMA's hospital evacuation system.
　Before a disaster, exercise scenarios should include dealing with the dilemma of patient evacuation versus shelter in place. If practical, i.e., there is warning before disaster strikes, consider sending home patients who can ambulate and keeping only the sickest under close clinical supervision. If the hospital leadership doesn't have time to ponder this kind of decision, it is made for the institution by default: shelter in place and prepare to take on mass casualities. Then evacuate when practical.
　The morgue, too, could be overrun…

Lesson 2—Stockpile Supplies

Adequate supplies are critical to managing a disaster event. Take inventory and refresh supplies periodically. Ensure that emergency provisions are stored in a place impenetrable to fire and flood, yet accessible. Non-perishable foods, linens, and personal care items are essential. Supplies should include the basics for surviving without power or running water for at least one week. This includes basic medicines and fully supplied first aid kits, portable generators and extension cords, fuel for the generators, buckets with thick red liner bags for toilets and other waste, hand sanitizer and other basic hygiene products, and paper towels for your personnel—multiplied times three or four, as others may seek refuge in your buildings, too.

Lesson 3—Family and Pets

If disaster is predictable, remember that workers have loved ones who could be in harm's way. So prepare to accommodate family inside your buildings if at all possible. And realize that pets are often considered part of the family. Plan for and allow workers to bring a pet to the building if a disaster is imminent (the pet owner must provide a carrier, food, medications, and care instructions for the duration). Many people will refuse to abandon their pets at home, so figure out how to accommodate the animals, especially if the community disaster plan does not deal with pet evacuation and shelter.

Lesson 4—Communications Systems

Have a modern communications system and make sure you are networked with the proper government authorities. Test the devices regularly. Mobile phone service may not work consistently during a catastrophic event; text messaging, however, operates off another network and might be of value—but not as a reliable communications system. Satellite phones have become common supplements to radio communication, although they may not be consistently dependable deep inside a building. Ham radio may be most reliable technologically, but perhaps impractical in some disaster situations because it is not a rapid form of communication. Ham radio depends on volunteer operators, and while they are a committed cohort, they too could be silenced in the disaster zone. And every hospital or healthcare organization should obtain a Government Emergency Telecommunications Service (GETS) card (at http://gets.ncs.gov/). The GETS card number will let you access a land line in disaster, with priority over other calls.

Lesson 5—Have a Back-Up Plan

The cavalry might not arrive. The cavalry might show up late. So if the disaster plan fails, there needs to be a back-up plan. There is ample evidence in recent disasters to illustrate this deadly serious point. There will likely be failures in key aspects of even the most sophisticated and thorough plans because there are so many variables in any given disaster. So if "Plan A" cannot be implemented for whatever reason, have "Plan

(continued)

B." This is especially important if (1) your emergency supplies, provisions, or auxiliary fuel are compromised or insufficient and (2) your evacuation plan cannot be executed as designed. Formal relationships with similar organizations, suppliers, and contracted "evacuators" should be established and carefully maintained.

Lesson 6—Don't Panic
Disaster comes in various forms and levels of intensity. It could be an isolated yet destructive fire that is extinguished in a matter of hours, or it could be as impactful as the total destruction of the Twin Towers in New York City in 2001. Leaders are leaders for a reason. They can manage difficult situations and keep their charges calm and motivated. Respect the danger, but don't let it consume you. How leaders comport themselves can set the tone for the staff's response to the disaster.

Lesson 7—Communicate
Some disasters are brief. Those are more common than 2005's Katrina or the Midwest floods during the summer of 2008. So having an established and regularly updated phone tree or e-mail outreach plan is important. Let the outside world, especially loved ones of workers who might be trapped, know what is happening. We all want to know what is going on when tragedy occurs.

In the event of a major disaster or tragedy on your organization's premises, communicate with the media and with others concerned about the situation. Do not shun the press. Don't let staff or security officers mistreat or disrespect even the most aggressive of reporters. If at all possible, give the media a designated location with electrical outlets, internet connectivity, and plenty of coffee. And periodically hold conferences with them en masse. Manage your message to the extent possible instead of leaving much to the imagination of a reporter who has to crank out a story whether or not the leader speaks to the media. Be truthful with the press, although, understandably, there are circumstances when incomplete information requires circumspection.

Lesson 8—Prepare for the Worst and Hope for the Best
Be prepared for heartache and let down. Know that despair will set in over the course of a disaster event. While there inevitably will be sadness and perhaps loss of life, the despair likely will come from a sense of not having control over the situation. Leaders are leaders, in part, because they can control a situation. Some major events come without manuals or steering wheels. So there are bound to be periods of helplessness.

In a disaster, one can expect a lack of cooperation even from some who are designated to support the organization. On the other hand, there may be unexpected angels that descend upon the site.

Expect a disaster to bring anxiety and tension. This may result not only from the complexity of the situation, but from fatigue. Sleep may be the last thing on one's mind during a multi-day event. But if time can possibly be spared, leaders and staff should rest in order to stay sharp—the organization depends on it.

Also expect that superiors, perhaps unaccustomed to disaster scenarios, may avoid the situation, either because of their geographic distance or their being otherwise ill-equipped. The result may be indecisiveness, or worse, uneducated direction. Know that this kind of failure can occur, and prepare to deal with it emotionally and tactically.

As a leader, expect to make periodic reports to superiors or other stakeholders, even if doing so seems frivolous during the heat of a major event. Not only can the organization retrospectively learn from your in-the-zone reports, they can also serve as important evidence when the inevitable audit or investigation occurs months later. After the disaster passes, no matter how devastating, the auditors, government investigators, or insurance agents will opine. They probably were not present during the event, and therefore might coldly evaluate the organization's performance. So prepare for and honestly deal with distasteful managerial issues such as impaired assets, inventory that mysteriously disappears at the time of the event, and AWOL employees.

Angels descend from unexpected places at unexpected times, but it is best not to plan on it.

Lesson 9—The Aftermath—A Sprint, Especially for Hospitals
After the disaster has come and gone, what remains of your institution will generally reveal what next steps in recovery are necessary. There may be physical damage to your buildings. There may be myriad impaired assets. Your employees and their loved ones may have suffered personally. The workforce may be depleted across the board or in specific functional areas. Interim facilities and outside help may be necessary, and immediately. The leadership must rally the organization by providing a game plan for returning to operation as quickly as possible, even if that means using temporary resources that otherwise wouldn't be considered in normal circumstances. Here is a checklist that can guide the plan for the first few weeks after the disaster:

The Business Side
- Do you know how much money you will lose from fully or partially interrupted operations?
- Do you know how long your hospital is financially viable given a reduction in or a complete loss of revenue?
- Have you worked out arrangements with bankers and debt holders regarding your situation?
- Do you know if your business interruption insurance has kicked in?
- Have your building damage insurance claims been addressed? Or FEMA claims?
- Have you reached out to local and national politicians for support?
- Have your suppliers agreed to support you in your short-term need? Or long-term need?
- Have you accounted for impaired or destroyed assets?

(continued)

The Clinical Side
- Do you have adequate relationships with other providers to coordinate community needs?
- Have you negotiated an agreement to operate interim facilities, if needed?
- Have you developed an operational plan to care for patients if you lose key clinical and support staff?
- Have you determined the impact on your medical staff and how the hospital should respond?
- Have you created a vision for restoration or replacement of clinical facilities?

Lesson 10—The Aftermath—A Marathon

Responding to the organization's needs after the disaster has damaged your human and physical infrastructure represents a difficult battle of competing interests. There are immediate priorities and there are long-term priorities. They are both so important that typical sequencing of activities is impractical. Addressing the organization's needs, both short term and long term, should be pursued simultaneously—and with equal vigor. Your long-term strategy could involve:

- Facility replacement or major renovation
- An entirely new business plan
- Seizing an opportunity to reconfigure or reinvent your organization
- A major campaign to gain support for the plan

At the end of the day, the successful leader will concurrently deal with the immediate post-disaster recovery while simultaneously launching the development of the long term-plan for not just viability, but excellence.

Donald R. Smithburg
Executive Associate Dean, College of Medicine.
Florida International University
Former CEO, Louisiana Charity Hospital System

AFTER THE DISASTER

Beware of post-crisis letdown. Expect some delayed stress reaction in your people who have been deeply involved. Depression, physical complaints, friction in routine work and at home, and irrational outbursts will occur. Don't be surprised when you discover these symptoms in yourself. You are not made of cast iron. If you were, you wouldn't have been able to manage this crisis.

Casualty assistance, survivor needs, and post-crisis considerations are three areas you will most likely neglect. However, these three have the greatest potential to create short- and long-term problems. Together, they present the greatest likelihood of destroying your achievements in managing the crisis.

Dr. Thomas Royer (2009), CEO of CHRISTUS Health, states that "debriefs of previous disaster response situations and debriefing regarding our response to this disaster have helped us ensure we are even better prepared for the next disaster." He also provides guiding principles for disaster leadership.

- Preparation is critical.
- Prepare for the worst.
- Stay focused and as calm as possible.
- Constant communication with all possible constituencies is key.
- Depend only on your internal team.

Managing the Aftermath of a Disaster with Mass Fatalities
- Assign a casualty assistance officer.
- Assign a mature, experienced chaplain as your personal representative to meet with the next of kin and care for their needs.
- Casualties are news, and this news travels rapidly. Your timely reactions will ease the burden on the next of kin.
- Provide for survivor needs.
- A public memorial service where participants can share their sense of pride and loss may help survivors.
- Assign the necessary security personnel to protect the privacy of survivors. Survivors are in no condition to talk to the media, investigators, or law enforcement officers. Do not make exceptions to this rule, except on the advice of a medical officer or chaplain.
- Coordinate and communicate with the organizations and individuals who want to help. Without supervision, they will create chaos.
- Anticipate a delayed stress reaction during the aftermath. Make sure medical officers and chaplains remain available to survivors and their families.

Source: Gilbert (1982).

Appendix 4.1: Thoughts on Preparing for an H1N1 Pandemic

Much planning took place in 2009 around the possible H1N1 (swine flu) outbreak. Many organizations planned to either significantly reduce or even suspend operations in the event that a large number of employees became ill with the virus. Employers urged staff who thought they were sick to stay home. School districts went so far as to shut entire schools when even a small handful of students became sick. Universities across the country made plans to teach classes via an online platform should faculty become infected with H1N1 or if large numbers of students became so ill that they were unable to attend classes.

All of these scenarios were plausible and made good sense to the general public. After all, why should sick employees go to work or students who have contracted H1N1 go to school and possibly infect others? Closing a business for a few days might result in a financial hardship to the owners and an inconvenience to customers, but in a short time, the firm will recover.

But what if a local hospital were to employ the same strategy? Imagine the outrage that would result if the local community hospital were to hang out a CLOSED sign on the emergency room doors because it had sent its doctors, nurses, and technicians home ill with the swine flu.

One of the most easily recognizable signs in the world is a blue rectangular sign with a capital white "H." In an event that disrupts the health or well-being of a community, the first place people generally go is to their local hospital. In 2001, during the time that anthrax-laced envelopes were delivered to a number of media outlets and two U.S. senators, hospital emergency departments were overrun with people who were convinced that they were infected and demanded treatment. Hospitals did not expect the large number of worried well to appear and seek care. The H1N1 situation posed a similar scenario. Virtually every daily news cycle had a story of people who had been diagnosed with swine flu and the attendant risk of death, particularly for vulnerable groups. Given the real and imagined fear associated with a possible swine flu pandemic, it was reasonable to ask if local hospitals were prepared for an event of this magnitude.

As we now know, fortunately the swine flu pandemic did not cause the widespread devastation we thought it might. But it's still wise to ask that same question: What do hospitals need to do to prepare for a pandemic such as H1N1?

First, the healthcare workforce must be first in line to receive the vaccine the moment it becomes available. Coupled with scrupulous hand washing, preventing the contraction of the flu is the first and best line of defense for the continuation of a robust healthcare delivery system.

Second, knowing that emergency departments would quickly be filled, hospital leaders should abandon the idea that the hospital is the only place patients can be treated. A regional emergency response network should be created, with the hospital at its center. Patients would be assessed (triaged) in the hospital and then, depending on their level of illness, be moved to alternate care sites or "bed-down" locations in gymnasiums, schools, or local malls. Local hospitals would use their professional staff, equipment, and supplies to resource the off-site location(s). If the pandemic was a relatively minor illness, as H1N1 was, the event would primarily cause minimal care cases, so patients at the bed-down sites could largely be managed by nurses and other paraprofessionals. It is incumbent on leaders of hospitals, local government, public safety, education, and business to have in place memoranda of understanding and other agreements before an actual pandemic occurs. The goal is to create a networked facility approach that prevents the local hospital from collapsing—thus maintaining the ability to care for affected communities.

Devastation in the wake of hurricanes Katrina and Rita showed us that the United States was fundamentally unprepared for major natural or man-made disasters. Even with three day's notice in advance of its arrival, Katrina clearly demonstrated the inability of public and private organizations to quickly and effectively protect people's lives and well-being. It is unarguable that the approximately 5,000 community hospitals in the United States must have the resilience to individually and/or collectively provide services to all who are affected by any future disaster regardless of its potential magnitude or the total number of individuals impacted. There is currently no easily administered and reliable method to accurately assess organizational resilience to disasters, and to use this information to expand the capacity of individual organizations to effectively respond to these events. In times of disaster, people immediately turn to their hospitals and other healthcare providers for care, information, and reassurance. These organizations simply must acquire the ability to withstand a severe jolt and continue to provide effective service.

Dr. Leonard Friedman PhD, MPA, MPH, FACHE
George Washington University

Part III
RECOVERY

CHAPTER 5

Recovery: The Good, the Bad, and the Ugly

Jane Kushma, PhD

So far, we have looked at the challenges associated with immediate response to a disaster and management of the crisis period. We now turn our attention to recovery from disaster, which is much more than restoring basic services or rebuilding damaged facilities and infrastructure. Of all four phases of disaster—mitigation, preparedness, response, and recovery—the recovery phase is the least researched and the most poorly understood. Moreover, few communities are truly prepared to implement recovery and reconstruction activities in the wake of a major disaster, and many businesses struggle to stay afloat.

A simple definition of *recovery* is picking up the pieces after a disaster and trying to return to some sense of normalcy. The term has been used synonymously with restoration, rebuilding, reconstruction, redevelopment, and rehabilitation. One of the most important lessons of disaster recovery is that if you invest some time thinking about how you will recover *before the disaster strikes*, this preparation will pay tremendous dividends in a disaster's aftermath. Anticipating demands, organizing resources, and determining a basic strategy increase efficiency and adaptability and reduce vulnerability.

The typical environment for recovery involves multiple and competing demands for restoration and rebuilding, intense pressure from a traumatized constituency to "return to normal," and a considerable drain on existing capacity caused by taking on new tasks while maintaining customary ones. These factors can powerfully influence the speed and quality of recovery.

In addition to the external challenges during recovery, organizations will face a multitude of internal demands, such as workforce issues, business resumption requirements, and economic threats. The good news is that these are demands you can anticipate and on which you can take action in advance of a disaster. While recovery is challenging, it also can present many opportunities. In particular, it can help you prepare for the next event.

DEFINING RECOVERY AND SUSTAINABILITY

Recovery has been linked to the concept of sustainability. According to the Brundtland Commission of the World Commission on Environment and Development (WCED 1987), *sustainable development* means meeting the needs of the present without compromising the ability of future generations to meet their own needs. Sustainable development, then, involves balancing social, environmental, and economic needs.

Sustainable communities

♦ make more efficient use of their land, including preventing development from encroaching upon floodplains, active fault zones, and other hazard areas;
♦ maintain social viability by balancing the competing needs of their citizens;
♦ maintain economic viability by keeping businesses out of high-risk areas or disaster proofing them if there is no practical way to relocate them; and
♦ maintain environmental sustainability by preserving natural systems and limiting environmental degradation.

Finally, resilience to disasters is an essential characteristic of sustainable communities (Godschalk 2003). While hazard forces might cause them to bend, resilient communities will not break. They can withstand major impacts without sustaining debilitating physical, social, or economic damage. *Resiliency* has also been used to describe ecological systems, in terms of their ability to recover from events such as droughts or changes in water supply.

Dennis Mileti (1999) defines resiliency in terms of the self-sufficiency of the community: "Local resiliency with respect to disasters means that a locale is able to withstand an extreme natural event without suffering devastating losses, damage, diminished productivity, or quality of life and without a large amount of assistance from outside the community." A resilient community, therefore, is a sustainable network of physical systems and human communities. Physical systems are the constructed components and natural environment of the community. Human communities are the social and institutional components of the community. Together, they make up the body and brains of the community. Sustainability is essential to survival in a "new normal." As you assess your vulnerability and disaster recovery needs, you must not do so in isolation. You need to understand not only your risks and the resources you can bring to bear, but also the broader community context and how it might affect your operations and client base.

EXTERNAL RECOVERY

Natural disasters exact a heavy toll on the United States. Each year, public and private entities spend billions of dollars on natural disaster recovery efforts. Disasters affect community life in several areas, including lifelines and infrastructure, housing, the economy, the environment, and social networks. Despite the resources devoted to recovery, many communities take a long time to bounce back, and some never completely recover. Even more disturbing, the U.S. Department of Labor estimates that "over 40 percent of businesses never reopen following a disaster. Of the remaining companies, at least 25 percent will close within two years. Over 60 percent of businesses confronted by a major disaster close by two years, according to the Association of Records Managers and Administration" (sbinformation. about.com, 2010).

Resources for Recovery

Institutional
Many resources exist to help you plan for your organization's survival and recovery after a disaster. The following online resources will help you identify the critical actions you need to take to recover from a disaster.

◆ **Open for Business: Disaster Planning Toolkit** (http://disastersafety.org/ resource/resmgr/pdfs/OpenForBusiness_new.pdf). This guide was prepared by the Institute for Business & Home Safety (IBHS). IBHS is a nonprofit initiative of the insurance industry to reduce the social and economic effects of natural disasters and other property losses by conducting research and advocating improved construction, maintenance, and preparation practices. The guide includes business continuity planning forms, a property protection checklist, and other disaster-planning guidance.

- **Operation Fresh Start** (http//www.freshstart.ncat.org/business.htm). This website provides additional resources to help plan for an effective recovery.

Community

Your local community typically will maintain an emergency operations plan (EOP), but this plan may or may not address community recovery. Talk with your local emergency manager to find out what is in place and how citizens and businesses will participate in the planning process. Your community also may have an organization that will coordinate voluntary efforts following a disaster (e.g., a local member organization of Voluntary Organizations Active in Disaster or VOAD). Some communities also have established business alliances to share information and coordinate efforts related to disaster. A local chapter of the Association of Contingency Planners (www.acp-international.com) may spearhead such an effort, or your local chamber of commerce may sponsor one.

For general recovery planning and guidance, check out the American Red Cross web page "Important Steps for Your Safe and Speedy Recovery" (www.redcross.org).

State and Federal Government

The Robert T. Stafford Disaster Relief and Emergency Assistance Act (Stafford Act) authorizes the president to issue major disaster or emergency declarations in response to catastrophes that overwhelm state and local governments.

Such declarations result in the distribution of federal aid to individuals and families, certain nonprofit organizations, and public agencies. Congress appropriates money to the Disaster Relief Fund (DRF), which is administered by the Federal Emergency Management Agency (FEMA) within the Department of Homeland Security (DHS), for disaster assistance authorized by the Stafford Act.

Federal disaster assistance is money or direct assistance to individuals, families, and businesses whose property has been damaged or destroyed and whose losses are not covered by insurance. It is meant to help with critical expenses that cannot be covered in other ways. The assistance is not intended to restore damaged property to its predisaster condition. While housing assistance funds are available through the FEMA Individuals and Households Program, most disaster assistance from the federal government is in the form of loans administered by the Small Business Administration (SBA).

FEMA also has a public assistance (PA) program that provides supplemental federal disaster grant assistance for debris removal, emergency protective measures, and the repair, replacement, or restoration of disaster-damaged, publicly owned facilities and the facilities of certain private nonprofit (PNP) organizations. The PA program also encourages protection of these damaged facilities from future disasters by offering assistance for hazard mitigation measures during recovery.

The following websites provide information about some of the main FEMA assistance programs.

◆ FEMA Public Assistance Program (www.fema.gov/government/grant/pa/index.shtm)
◆ FEMA Individual Assistance Program (www.fema.gov/individual/grant.shtm)
◆ ESF #14 Long-Term Community Recovery (www.fema.gov/rebuild/ltcr)

In addition to federal assistance available from FEMA, the SBA has a significant disaster assistance program. SBA can make federally subsidized loans to repair or replace homes, personal property, or businesses that sustained damages from a disaster that are not covered by insurance. These disaster loans can be divided into three categories:

1. Home disaster loans to homeowners and renters to repair or replace disaster-related damages to home or personal property
2. Business physical disaster loans to business owners to repair or replace disaster-damaged property, including inventory, and supplies
3. Economic injury disaster loans, which provide capital to small businesses and small agricultural cooperatives to assist them through the disaster recovery period

For many individuals, the SBA disaster loan program is the primary form of disaster assistance. To learn how to apply for SBA disaster loan assistance, visit www.sba.gov/services/disasterassistance/index.html.

Finally, FEMA provides a guide that includes brief descriptions and contact information for all federal programs that provide disaster recovery assistance to eligible applicants. You can access this guide online at www.fema.gov/pdf/rebuild/ltrc/recoveryprograms229.pdf.

Additional information on the financial aspects of disasters may be found in Chapters 6 and 7.

IMPORTANCE OF HAZARD MITIGATION

The Multihazard Mitigation Council of the National Institute of Building Sciences (2005) published the report "Natural Hazard Mitigation Saves: An Independent Study to Assess the Future Savings from Mitigation Activities." This report was the result of a congressionally mandated independent study, commissioned by FEMA, which began in 2000. The study was based on a detailed work plan developed by a team of experts in various aspects of hazards mitigation and benefit assessment from the Multihazard Mitigation Council Board and concluded that natural hazards mitigation is cost-effective. On average, one dollar spent by FEMA on hazard mitigation saves the nation about four dollars in future benefits. In addition, grants provided by FEMA to mitigate the effects of hurricanes, tornadoes, floods, and earthquakes between 1993 and 2003 were expected to save more than 220 lives and prevent about 4,700 injuries over approximately 50 years.

INTERNAL RECOVERY

We have looked at disasters and their aggregate effects. We now want to turn our attention to more specific challenges that you and your employees may face as a result of a disaster and what you can do about them.

Workforce Issues

Clearly, a disaster can disrupt your normal business operations. Your physical location, your employees' homes, or both may experience damage. How will you address these concerns while attempting to minimize suffering, reduce losses, and resume operations as quickly as possible? You may want to build some of the following resources into your current planning efforts.

Employee Assistance
The Weyerhaeuser (2005) guide documents innovative strategies, best practices, and tactics for helping employees. It includes checklists, processes for case-management advocacy, and streamlined claims-processing forms.

Children and Pets
Children and pets are important family members who may need special attention following a disaster. You can provide a critical service to your employees by helping them understand some of the typical reactions to a disaster they might expect from their children and where they can get more information. Disaster preparedness for pets is an important, although often overlooked, need.

Child Care
Healthcare facilities often shelter families and children of employees. Their care must be age-specific, with appropriate activities and tasks assigned. Age-specific

guidelines for providing employee child care can be found in the FEMA guide *Helping Children Cope with a Disaster* (www.fema.gov/pdf/library/children.pdf).

Pet Care

Realizing that employees and staff may refuse to report to duty if their pets are at risk, many healthcare organizations provide, and some accrediting agencies require, the provision of pet care. The following documents provide useful planning assistance for this important service.

- FEMA, *Information for Pet Owners* (www.fema.gov/plan/prepare/animals.shtm)
- Disaster preparedness quiz from the Humane Society of the United States (www.hsus.org/hsus_field/hsus_disaster_center/resources/disaster_preparedness_quiz.html)
- Centers for Disease Control and Prevention, *Protect Your Pets in an Emergency* (http://emergency.cdc.gov/disasters/petprotect.asp)

Mental Health Recovery

The emotional toll of a disaster can be overwhelming. Being aware of available community counseling resources and encouraging your employees to use them, including any employee assistance program contract services you may use, can reduce distress and facilitate recovery. The American Psychological Association provides an online resource that may help you understand the emotional impacts of disasters, and what to do about them: *Managing Traumatic Stress: Tips for Recovering from Disasters and Other Traumatic Events* (www.apa.org/helpcenter/recovering-disasters.aspx).

Operations

Planning for effective recovery of operations is crucial for healthcare facilities. Remaining operational is expected, and it's critical for maintaining the trust of the community. Operational aspects benefiting from predisaster recovery planning include

- facility function and stability;
- ability to keep equipment operational and safe;
- availability and renewability of supplies; and
- systems needs, such as
  - administration and management,
  - information management,
  - communications, and
  - emergency preparedness and management.

Market Share Challenges

Following a significant disaster, the healthcare facility may face unanticipated market share challenges. Following Hurricane Katrina, the New Orleans area population decreased from a pre-event level of 485,000 to an estimated population in September 2008 of 272,000—just 56 percent of the original population (RAND Corporation 2006).

The Greater New York Hospital Association developed an excellent tool, the "Recovery Checklist for Hospitals After a Disaster" (Exhibit 5.1). This internal tool, intended to assist facilities in maintaining a safe environment of care, identifies potential issues for review after a disaster in assessing the status of operations.

Additional resources for recovery include the following:

- Department of Homeland Security: Ready Business (www.ready.gov/business/index.html)
- FEMA: *Emergency Management Guide for Business and Industry* (www.fema.gov/business/guide/index.shtm)

Exhibit 5.1 Recovery Checklist for Hospitals After a Disaster

- Access and egress
  - Building(s)
  - Electrical systems
  - Facilities and engineering
  - Waste management
  - Water systems
- Communications: Internal and external
- Clinical services
  - Dialysis
  - Dietary
  - Emergency department
  - Infection control
  - Information technology/ medical records
  - Laboratory
  - Morgue
  - Pharmacy
  - Radiology
  - Security
  - Surgical services
  - Sterile supply systems
- Emergency preparedness and management
- Equipment and supplies
- Management and administration
- Personnel
- Vendors

Source: Greater New York Hospital Association. "Recovery Checklist for Hospitals After A Disaster." ML-236. October 26 2006. Web: http://www.nyc.gov/html/doh/downloads/pdf/bhpp/bhpp-hospital-tools-checklist.pdf

---

CHAPTER 6

Financial Planning for Catastrophic Events

G. Edward Tucker, Jr., CPA, CMC
Calvin Foster (Insurance Section)

Many hospital chief financial officers (CFOs) falsely assume that their role in planning for and responding to catastrophic events is limited to maintaining proper insurance for the institution. Nothing could be further from the truth, as this chapter explains. Catastrophic events can significantly impair a healthcare business, and if the CFO fails to fully participate in the planning, these events can cause bond defaults and even bankruptcy.

Financial planning for catastrophic events involves the following activities. Each of these activities is discussed in this chapter (see Exhibit 6.1).

- Allocate an adequate budget for disaster planning.
- Accumulate enough days cash on hand.
- Arrange a line of credit.
- Get the right insurance coverage.
- Minimize cost by advance planning.
- Form a claims-filing team and provide training.
- Set aside funds for employee financial assistance.
- Plan for the aftereffects.

Exhibit 6.1 Checklist for Catastrophic Event Financial Planning

- Allocate an adequate budget for disaster planning.
- Accumulate enough days cash on hand.
- Arrange a line of credit.
- Get the right insurance coverage.
- Minimize cost by advance planning.
- Form a claims-filing team and provide training.
- Set aside funds for employee financial assistance.
- Plan for the aftereffects.

ALLOCATE AN ADEQUATE BUDGET FOR DISASTER PLANNING

Your healthcare organization likely has a budget allocated for disaster events, although these funds may be scattered among various functional budgets. Under *responsibility accounting*—a system that relies on department managers to control and monitor their unit's expenses and revenues—only one person is in charge of budget management for the department. Each of these managers likely allocates funds for catastrophic or disaster events for his or her unit—which explains why the disaster planning budget is not combined. This practice is acceptable, assuming that the budgeting process is coordinated among the various units to ensure that funds are allocated in each department's budget.

Following is a list of items to include in the catastrophe budget (see Exhibit 6.2):

- The appropriate amount of days cash on hand
- Insurance
- Information systems and business recovery
- Security
- Disaster equipment and supplies
- Training and drills
- Other

Not all of these items are dedicated to disaster response and preparedness, but they are important for the unit's daily functioning. Disasters are infrequent, but the likelihood that they will happen increases the need for a comprehensive disaster budget. These budget items are discussed throughout this chapter.

Exhibit 6.2 Budget Items for Catastrophic Event Financial Planning

- Days cash on hand
- Insurance
- Information systems and business recovery
- Security
- Disaster equipment and supplies
- Training and drills
- Other

ACCUMULATE ENOUGH DAYS CASH ON HAND

Days cash on hand (DCOH) is used by financial analysts to evaluate the financial health of organizations, including healthcare entities. Essentially, DCOH is a measure of how many days the organization could operate if it earns no revenue and has to use its cash reserves. This measure is key in disaster planning because a catastrophe can severely interrupt the revenue stream and cash flow.

Reasons for cash flow disruption during a disaster include the following:

- The organization is unable to provide and bill for services.
- Physicians are absent and thus cannot admit or refer patients to any of the organization's services, such as the hospital, nursing home, rehabilitation facility, and home care agency.
- Third-party payers cannot receive and process claims.
- Patients' resources are either tied up or spent, making them unable to pay their health insurance premiums or copays.

In addition, a catastrophe causes expenses to rise, either temporarily or for a long period, because it requires much more than what the available functions and resources can handle. This extra expense drains DCOH. Here are some of the sources of this higher cost, during and after a disaster:

- Extra manpower, water, food, drugs, supplies, transportation, fuel, security, cleanup, equipment (e.g., generators, beds) rentals and repairs, and other necessities
- Overtime pay and use of agency nursing to cope with high patient demand and personnel shortage

- Preparing and filing insurance and FEMA claims, including staff time, consultants, and attorneys
- Maintenance and/or repair of overloaded, damaged, or compromised information systems and other electronic connections

In this environment of reduced revenue and increased expenses, having enough DCOH is imperative. A few weeks after a disaster, an organization hit by a disaster may have easily spent 60 to 75 days of its DCOH. Rebuilding this cash reserve can take years. Thus, the starting DCOH should be at or above the median for an organization rated as "investment grade." If it is, the DCOH level is itself a form of insurance.

DCOH is calculated as follows:

$$\textbf{DCOH} = \frac{\text{Cash + Marketable securities}}{(\text{Annual operating expenses} - \text{Depreciation and amortization})/365}$$

The numerator of this ratio calculates the amount of cash or "near cash" that the organization has. The denominator calculates one day of cash-type operating expenses; note that depreciation and amortization do not consume cash. The audited financial statements provide the numbers needed for this calculation.

If the organization has bondholders or other debtors, its debt covenants likely have a minimum DCOH—*that is, the lowest agreed-upon cash reserve level.* If the DCOH falls below this level, the organization may be considered in "default" of the debt covenant, which will require the organization to take corrective actions that are agreeable to the bondholders or other debtors. Usually, the minimum DCOH is within the 75–90 days range; however, the organization should maintain much more cash than this to protect itself from default. More important, a high reserve level ensures that the organization continues to operate and does not run low on cash.

The median DCOH range for hospitals rated "A" or higher is 150 to 180 days; for those rated "AA," the range is 180 to 200 days. For planning purposes, executives and managers should consult with the bond-rating agencies (e.g., Moody's, Fitch, Standard & Poor's) and the organization's bond insurer, if any. Also critical in this process is your own estimate of the appropriate DCOH. Exhibit 6.3 is a worksheet for estimating the impact of a disaster on the organization's cash position.

The next steps in financial planning for catastrophic events are discussed in the following sections.

Exhibit 6.3 Worksheet for Estimating the Cash Impact of a Catastrophe

	Length of Business Interruption		
	10 days	30 days	90 days
One day's cash operating expenses (from denominator of DCOH calculation)			
Multiply by number of days of interrupted cash flow	× 10	× 30	× 90
Cash Drain for Normal Expenses			
Extra expenses			
• Labor			
• Water			
• Food			
• Drugs			
• Supplies			
• Transportation			
• Security			
• Equipment rental and repair			
• Contract cleanup and repair			
• Other			
• Other			
• Other			
Cash Drain for Extra Expenses			
Total Cash Drain			

ARRANGE A LINE OF CREDIT

The best time to set up a line of credit is when credit is not needed. If the organization is fiscally sound, banks will compete for the opportunity to provide it with a line of credit, even if the funds will be used only for disaster recovery. But what bank in its right mind would lend money to an organization impaired by a disaster? One that values a long-term relationship with that organization is the answer.

Banks always want collateral from debtors. Here are some sources of collateral:

◆ Marketable securities that are not cashed in because of unrealized losses
◆ Pledge of insurance proceeds to be received for business interruption or physical damage (with permission of your bondholder trustee)
◆ Equipment or other assets not previously pledged

But if the bank truly values the relationship with the organization, it may offer an unsecured line of credit.

The organization's bond covenants may require it to obtain bondholder approval of such borrowing. If the line of credit is set up ahead of time or before an actual need arises, bondholders may welcome the influx of cash to help prevent the deterioration of fiscal operations. The organization may be able to pledge as collateral any expected advances from payers such as Medicare or Blue Cross to pay down some or all of the line of credit. Keep in mind that payer advances are short-term funds and may even need to be repaid before the line of credit is repaid.

As part of the financial planning for catastrophic events, arranging for a line of credit ahead of time is advantageous. In the event of a disaster, the organization can invoke the line of credit with negotiated rates and with only a minimum delay.

GET THE RIGHT INSURANCE COVERAGE

Calvin Foster

Healthcare organizations face two general types of exposures or vulnerabilities for which they need to be insured:

1. *Physical damage,* which is easily identifiable
2. *Business interruption,* which results in loss of income and profit caused by a covered event. The amount of loss is hard to identify and calculate, and this interruption can have a longer term and larger financial effect than the physical damage.

Valuing the Physical Plant

An understanding of valuation for insurance purposes is critical. Accounting or book value of the plant and its physical assets has no relevance in insurance valuation. If the book value is used, the organization could end up vastly under-insured. In the insurance contract, valuation is typically developed on the basis of replacement cost, which is defined as "the cost to replace or repair with like kind and quality with no deduction for depreciation. Actual cash value (ACV) is replacement cost less depreciation. Depreciation is physical depreciation, *not* the accumulated depreciation reflected in the book values on the financial statements.

Physical plant valuation is performed by obtaining an appraisal of current replacement cost—that is, determining what it would cost to build this facility at today's prices. The same process is used to assess the values of equipment and other contents of the plant. However, consideration must be given to the fact that some equipment may be outdated and will need to be replaced by newer models or more recent technology. Insurance coverage of the physical plant and assets should address these types of situations.

Estimating the Business Interruption

Business interruption is a complex insurance coverage, written with different coverage forms or provisions and limitations that either expand or limit the recovery from the standard forms. This type of insurance may be purchased separately or added on as an endorsement to property insurance. Under this insurance, the organization must specify what will be covered, such as property and loss of income, and must show proof that the disruption led to its inability to conduct business. Estimating the business interruption for insurance purposes involves these steps:

1. Determine the dollar values of items to be insured.
2. Identify the organization's specific exposures.

Determine the dollar values of items to be insured.
This first step may be performed by using a business interruption worksheet. This worksheet helps in forecasting the earnings that may be lost during and after an interruption as well as the cost of continuing operations during this period. Many different forms of worksheets are available; however, they follow the same basic format and include these elements:

1. Estimated revenue for the period
2. Deduction for noncontinuing expenses, such as supplies, utilities, and taxes on revenue
3. Continuing payroll, which includes key employees and other personnel and may be excluded completely from the calculation

The business interruption recovery period can be adjusted to reflect the specific period of recovery, such as 6 months, 12 months, or 15 months. If the recovery period is 6 months, then the valuation is 50 percent of the annual values, 15 months is 125 percent of annual values, and so on.

Business Interruption Values Worksheet
(Part of the Application or Update Process)

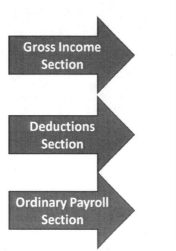

Gross Income Section

Deductions Section

Ordinary Payroll Section

Details below

BIV Worksheet – Gross Income Section

	Actual Value for 12 Months Ending	Estimated Value for 12 Months Ending
A. GROSS INCOME		
1. In-patient services	$ -	$ -
2. Out-patient services	$ -	$ -
3. Emergency ward	$ -	$ -
4. Grants and research contracts	$ -	$ -
5. School(s) - Tuition fees and other income	$ -	$ -
6. Commisions and/or rents from leased departments	$ -	$ -
7. Cafeteria, gift shop, bookstore	$ -	$ -
8. Ambulance	$ -	$ -
9. All other income (excluding donations and contributions)	$ -	$ -
TOTAL GROSS INCOME	$ -	$ -

Identify the organization's specific exposures.

This second step entails determining the organization's unique exposures or vulnerabilities in an event of a disaster. Healthcare organizations share similar exposures, such as loss to physical plant and business interruption; however, each organization has its own unique exposures against which it must insure. These exposures vary depending on the type and size of operation and the location. For example, a

BIV Worksheet – Deductions Section

	Actual Value for 12 Months Ending	Estimated Value for 12 Months Ending
B. DEDUCT COST OF		
1. Contractual adjustments, bad debts and free services	$ -	$ -
2. Supplies and materials	$ -	$ -
3. Merchandise sold	$ -	$ -
4. Services purchased from outsiders	$ -	$ -
5. Ordinary payroll - **Do not deduct wages of anyone under guaranteed annual compensation contracts or anyone retained during suspension of your operation.**	$ -	$ -
6. Compensation insurance premiums, Social Security, Unemployment Insurance and Other Charges allocated to Ordinary Payroll	$ -	$ -
7. Other non-continuing expenses (explain)	$ -	$ -
TOTAL DEDUCTIONS	$ -	$ -
ANNUAL VALUE FOR GROSS EARNINGS COVERAGE	$ -	$ -

BIV Worksheet – Ordinary Payroll Section

	Actual Value for 12 Months Ending	Estimated Value for 12 Months Ending
C. ORDINARY PAYROLL COVERAGE *If Ordinary Payroll coverage is desired please fill out the following information:*		
1. Ordinary Payroll (Section B-5 above)	$ -	$ -
2. Compensation insurance premiums, Social Security, Unemployment Insurance and Other Charges allocated to Ordinary Payroll (Section B-6 above)	$ -	$ -
3. Select the number of days that you would like to cover your ordinary payroll (Use the drop down box to select 30, 60, 90, 120, 270, or 360 days)	-	-
VALUE FOR ORDINARY PAYROLL COVERAGE	$ -	$ -

hospital located on the Gulf Coast is exposed to high winds and flooding because of the seasonal hurricanes in that area. Similarly, an operation in San Francisco is vulnerable to earthquakes. These two types of exposures do not apply to facilities in Minnesota.

These exposures contribute to business interruption and thus must be accounted for when structuring the organization's insurance coverage.

An organization's insurance deductible is the part of the risk it assumes. Deductibles for organizations located in areas with few catastrophes are usually consistent throughout all the risks the organization insures; however, deductibles for organizations in catastrophe-prone areas vary by exposure and can be much higher for certain risks.

Premiums are driven by the exposures. Naturally, premiums for hospitals in disaster-prone areas are higher than premiums for organizations located elsewhere.

Selecting the Coverage Forms or Provisions

Many forms of coverage or provisions are available to healthcare organizations. The following is a short list of the key provisions, but the organization should consider other forms and pay close attention to the exclusions.

- *All risk.* Note that a true all-risk coverage does not exist because all forms present certain exclusions. Many carriers provide different all-risk coverage forms and some of these are broader than others. For properties with large insured values, a *manuscript policy,* which offers the broadest coverage, is sometimes developed. The wording of a manuscript policy is specific to the insured property.
- *Replacement cost.* This provision replaces or repairs the property with like kind and quality and does not include a deduction for depreciation.
- *Blanket.* True blanket coverage allows you to place your limits where needed at the time of loss. Blanket coverage is preferred when insuring two or more buildings or two or more items (buildings and contents). For example, say you have ten buildings with a value of $1 million each, with a blanket building and contents limit of $10 million. You have a total loss at one of the buildings and determine that it will take $1,250,000 to replace the building, rather than just $1 million. You pull the $1,250,000 from the blanket limit ($10 million) and apply it to the total loss.
- *Agreed amount.* Most insurance contracts require the insurance coverage to be a certain percentage of the property's total value. The standard is to insure 80 percent of the total value, but the insured value can be 90 percent or even 100 percent. This provision is referred to as the *coinsurance clause.* If the hospital chooses a coverage amount less than what the coinsurance clause requires, the insurer could reduce any claim payment by the same percentage of the deficiency. For example, if the property is worth $100,000 and the coinsurance clause is 80 percent, the hospital is required to carry $80,000 coverage. If it only carries $60,000, which is 25 percent less than the clause stipulates, the

insurance company could reduce claims payments by 25 percent.

- An agreed-amount endorsement deletes the coinsurance clause and is set on the basis of an agreement on the value insured. The agreed-amount endorsement eliminates the possibility of a coinsurance penalty provision. To attach this endorsement, the carrier requires that the property be insured to full replacement cost.

Here are points to remember in selecting insurance provisions for business interruption coverage:

- Business interruption loss is triggered by the direct damage to the physical property insured or loss of the asset insured.
- Make sure that the business interruption policy is suited to the organization's operations, as this insurance form provides a wide array of loss-of-income coverage.
- Ordinary payroll or "nonessential employees" cost is deducted but can be added back for a specific period of time. The business interruption insurance form allows the organization to exclude payroll for all employees except managers, executives, and certain personnel. This is called *ordinary payroll*. Coverage for ordinary payroll can be added, however, for 30, 60, or 90 days for a premium add-on.
- "Extra expense" should be included in business interruption coverage. Extra expense coverage pays for the additional spending necessary to continue business functions in the event that a covered item (e.g., plant, equipment) sustains damage and disrupts normal business. The extra expense category can cover costs such as setting up temporary phone systems or offices, cleanup, and repairs.
- "Extended period of income" is an important but often overlooked provision. The business interruption period of indemnity is *from* the time the loss occurs *to* the time the business reopens. Often, however, after an interruption, the business may reopen but not operate at the same level it did before sustaining the loss. Extended period of indemnity provides the organization a specific length of time after the period of indemnity has ended to return its operation to a pre-catastrophe level of functioning. This extended period can last a full year.

Customizing Insurance to Fit the Specific Operation

The insurance structure should not focus on the small, day-to-day exposures to loss but on the big, catastrophic loss—whether man-made (e.g., arson, terrorist attack) or natural (e.g., tornado, flood, hurricane). Well-structured insurance can handle both man-made and natural losses. Coverage should reflect exposures to natural events, such as severe storms, wind, and earthquakes. Some facilities that are located in natural catastrophe–prone areas (such as the Gulf Coast) have coverage limitations imposed by insurers or regulators. But this provision should be built into the insurance coverage, and the limits should normally be adequate to cover loss.

Property deductibles are part of the risk the organization is assuming, and they vary according to the organization's appetite for risk. Deductibles for facilities located in non-catastrophe-prone areas are usually in the same, reasonable range; for those in catastrophe-prone areas, the deductibles vary and are usually sizable. Premiums are also driven by exposures. As can be expected, premiums are higher in catastrophe-prone areas than in other locations. Measuring and understanding the financial impact of exposures and its accompanying deductible and premiums are a must for personnel in charge of designing organization-specific insurance coverage.

Exhibit 6.4 sums up the key points in getting the right insurance coverage for disaster planning purposes.

Exhibit 6.4 Points to Remember in Insuring for Catastrophic Events

- The organization's insurance coverage should be specific to its needs.
- Identify the organization's exposures, which are driven by the operation's type and size, as well as by its location.
- Determine the dollar value of loss to the physical plant and the loss from business interruption. Use worksheets as necessary.
- Learn the basics of coverage forms or provisions and limitations.
- Pay close attention to what is not covered (exclusions) and what is covered. Under the all-risk form, what is not excluded is covered.
- Coverage for facilities located in a catastrophe-prone area is often limited. These limits should be adequate to cover the organization's loss following a disaster.
- Property deductible must be measured to ensure it fits the organization's appetite for risk.
- Premiums are driven by exposures. Properties in catastrophe-prone areas are charged a higher premium than those in other areas.
- Insurance records must be complete, and backup copies should be stored on-site and off-site.
- Lines of communication—agent to broker, broker to carrier, and carrier to organization—must be open and established ahead of time. In the event of a disaster, the organization should notify the carrier as soon as possible or give the carrier advance notice if possible.

Claims Planning

From an insurance and risk management perspective, proper claims planning can make the process run smoother and bring the claim to conclusion more quickly. Claims processes may vary from one organization to the next, but here is a general guideline for advance planning:

1. Review the insurance policy language with the broker or a consultant to ensure that the coverage is appropriate for the needs and realities of the organization.
2. Require the insurance carrier to appoint an adjuster who will specifically handle claims from the organization. The adjuster may be someone referred by the broker or a consultant, and he or she should be well versed in the type of exposures faced by the organization and the types of claims that result from those exposures.
3. Establish clear lines of communication among a representative from the organization, the broker, the adjuster, and other parties involved in reporting or handling claims from the organization.
4. Conduct a pre-loss meeting (with the broker taking the lead) with the underwriter, designated adjuster, and claims personnel. Among the items to discuss at this meeting are the details of the coverage, limitations, loss-adjustment parameters, and general and specific expectations.

MINIMIZE COST BY ADVANCE PLANNING

The cost of a catastrophe is measured not only in dollars spent but also in exposure of patients and staff to risk. In the aftermath of Hurricane Katrina, for example, ugly allegations arose about the supposed inadequate planning and action by management and staff of hospitals and nursing home facilities that allegedly caused patients' suffering and even death. Much of this risk can be mitigated by advance planning, supported by strong financial planning.

Hospitals are perceived as small, self-supporting "cities" that can survive on their own in an event of a disaster. The city analogy holds true for a short period, but over time, the hospital's dependence on utility services, logistical supply chain, telecommunications, road access, police and fire departments, and other public safety services becomes apparent. In a widespread catastrophe, such as that brought on by Hurricane Katrina, public and private services are overwhelmed or damaged and thus are not reliable. Hospitals must plan for the loss of these critical support services.

An integrated operational and financial disaster plan prepares the organization for the following contingencies after a disaster:

- Inadequate or loss of water supply
- Shortage of food
- Electrical power outage
- Shortage of fuel
- Shortage of essential medical and other supplies
- Patient transfers

Each of these aftereffects is discussed in this section to serve as a starting point for your team's own financial planning efforts.

Inadequate Water Supply

Loss or poor quality of water can be the most disruptive consequence of a catastrophe, especially for a hospital. Water is used in almost every aspect of operations, from customer and staff comfort to clinical care to sanitation. In a disaster that cuts off the water supply, a hospital competes with other institutions in the area, not to mention the population at large, for available clean water. Buying water bottles and ice is not only expensive but also inefficient, and there is no guarantee that they can be easily obtained, as people tend to hoard water for their own use.

Some medical services, such as dialysis, rely on pure water. Dialysis patients are put in danger without their treatments, and these treatments are impossible without water. Hand-washing—one of the simplest safeguards against hospital-acquired infections—is impossible without water. Laundry, housekeeping, and food services are also on hold, as well as patient and staff showers and flushing toilets. Lack of water can quickly turn a hospital into an unsanitary and uncomfortable place.

Water outage must be included in financial planning, and capital expenditure should be allocated to ensure proper operating agreements are made. For example, water delivery in tanker trucks or trailers may be made with the local government or the National Guard. Alternatively, as one hospital has done, a deep well may be dug on the hospital property and a water tower that holds supply for a certain number of days may be built. The well and tower may be integrated with the local government's system, and the local government may be contracted to manage the supply, including cycling the water through the system to keep it fresh. The capital expenditure and operating agreement will require financial planning.

Shortage of Food

Food supply for healthcare organizations is a "just-in-time" item—that is, it is delivered as needed. Because of this practice, not much food is stored in the facility. Power outages are common in disasters, and without power, stored (frozen) food spoils. Regular suppliers in the area are unreliable in such conditions, as they too are hit by the same catastrophe.

The best plan against such shortage is to make arrangements with alternate suppliers who are located some distance from the hospital location. This way, when the area is struck by disaster, the alternate supplier may not be affected and can be relied on to make needed deliveries. Note that this plan is not foolproof as roads may be closed; however, early planning allows you and the supplier to discuss alternative forms of delivery.

The financial plan should include a trade credit arrangement with an alternate supplier. When prearranged, this agreement may allow sales-tax exemption and provide other financial incentives.

Electrical Power Outage

All hospitals are required to have emergency generators that kick on instantly when normal power goes out. However, most hospitals' emergency generators are not equipped for the full, around-the-clock operations of a hospital, so emergency power is limited to certain critical areas. Only equipment plugged into designated emergency power outlets ("red plugs") will work. Often, HVAC systems will not work.

Generators require shutdown and maintenance after a number of hours of operation. They also fail—sometimes during periods when they are most needed. Even if the facility has other standby generators, it is not likely they would be able to handle the high power demand of the entire facility, including HVAC systems, especially if the outage extends over days or weeks. Without reliable electrical power, the hospital cannot operate effectively, efficiently, and safely for very long.

The financial manager helps plan for backup electrical power. Typically this will involve a contract with one or more companies to supply generators on trailers that can be brought in before or after an event in case the hospital's backup generator fails or needs maintenance.

Electronic equipment fails when it overheats. Therefore, financial and operational disaster planning should consider the need for generating capacity in areas of critical patient care and information systems equipment, such as surgery, radiology, emergency department, and patient care units. The generating capacity may need to provide enough power to run the air conditioning and ventilation system. This can be expensive.

One hospital contracted with the local power company to build and maintain a 7.5 megawatt diesel-powered electrical generating facility on the hospital's campus. The facility is owned by the hospital and is leased to the power company; the power company, in turn, leases the generators from a third party and maintains and tests them. The generators are hooked to both the hospital's and power company's grids, but first priority goes to the hospital in time of need. The power company bills the hospital each month for maintaining the capability, and if the generators are dispatched to the power company grid, the hospital receives a credit for energy sold to the grid. This arrangement took significant planning by engineering and finance personnel.

Shortage of Fuel

In time of disaster, the hospital's generator capacity must be directly fueled on the hospital premises, creating an extra logistical problem in time of disaster, as fuel supplies may be short. The fuel logistics are complicated further by competition for fuel from the community, National Guard, ambulance services, employees, etc.

Financial planning for catastrophes should include a budget for bulk purchase of fuel (diesel and gasoline), to be used for the hospital's generators, vehicles, ambulances, and other equipment; this fuel may also be used for employee vehicles if needed. One county-owned hospital teamed up with the county government to buy an independent fuel wholesale business that was moving its depot elsewhere. This purchase now enables the county, the hospital, and its ambulance service to store fuel in bulk and provides fuel for its needs during both normal and emergency operations. Buying fuel in bulk and in advance also saves the organization money.

Shortage of Essential Medical and Other Supplies

Clearly, disaster situations increase the demand for emergency and nonemergency medical services and thus use up existing supplies. Supply chain management is typically the direct responsibility of the CFO, and part of this role is to look for efficient and cost-effective ways to replenish supplies. Joining a group purchasing organization—an entity that takes advantage of its members' purchasing power—is one way financial planners can find alternate suppliers and get big discounts from vendors. As mentioned before, these arrangements must be made in advance to prevent shortages of necessary supplies in the middle of a catastrophe.

Patient Transfers

Transferring patients to another facility, because hospital operations have been crippled by a catastrophe, can be costly. Ground and air ambulance services will most likely want a guaranteed payment for transfers. But when patients' lives are at risk, no one will have the time to negotiate transfer prices and payment terms or "shop around" for better rates. Therefore, the costs and logistics of patient transfers following a disaster must be identified, analyzed, developed, and agreed upon before the actual need arises.

Disaster financial planners should consider many factors, including the following:

♦ Rates, reliability record, on-board equipment, and location of multiple ground and air ambulance services
♦ Costs to relieve transfer crews if they have to work an extended period
♦ Type of aircraft (Fixed-wing aircraft is less expensive than rotary-wing aircraft; a fleet that uses both types is cost-effective.)

FORM AND TRAIN A CLAIMS-FILING TEAM

Filing insurance claims and applying for FEMA (Federal Emergency Management Agency) reimbursement and grants are time-consuming and involved processes that require detailed documentation. Those responsible for filing these claims must be given appropriate training. But first, the organization must form a claims-filing team made up of the following members:

♦ CFO
♦ Risk manager
♦ Controller
♦ Reimbursement manager
♦ Director of engineering and maintenance
♦ Other department managers (for plant damage and business interruption purposes)
♦ External professionals
  • insurance agent
  • attorney
  • forensic accountants
  • cost report specialist
  • consultants, as needed

Conflicts of interest may arise when doing business with outside professionals. For example, many attorneys practice insurance defense. The organization's attorney may be ineligible to be part of the claims team if he or she has dealings with the organization's insurer.

The entire team should review the financial plan so that all members are aware of its contents; this review should be done at least once annually. Training the team on FEMA and insurance rules may entail a mixture of both internal and external instructions.

SET ASIDE FUNDS FOR EMPLOYEE FINANCIAL ASSISTANCE

Employees often go through difficulties following a catastrophe. Some lose all their belongings, and some have no one to turn to for help—financial or otherwise. The hospital or its foundation (if any) should plan for such an outcome, extending assistance to employees who have short-term or long-term need.

A fundraiser, formal or informal, is a good way to amass funds for employee assistance. Employees, vendors, the community, local businesses, and other institutions in the area are potential donors. A hospital in another state might "adopt" your hospital to raise funds, while your hospital may do the same for that institution. The most important element in this fundraising is to do it before the need arises, especially for facilities in catastrophe-prone areas.

Criteria for financial assistance must be established to prevent an imbalance in disbursement and to discourage people from taking advantage. The following criteria may be applied:

- The disaster must have caused the need; proof of loss should be shown.
- Long-term versus short-term needs may require different criteria.
- The amount of aid given depends on the employee's need, income level, and received insurance proceeds (if any).
- Aid is not indefinite; it has specific start and end dates. Otherwise, some assistance may be viewed as an entitlement or an expected benefit of employment.

Keep in mind that financial assistance may cause dissent among employees, specifically if the criteria are perceived as unfair or favoring one group over another. One hospital contracted with the United Way to adjudicate claims to ensure confidentiality and objectivity.

PLAN FOR THE AFTEREFFECTS

Recognize that a catastrophe may affect the community's economy for an extended period, such as in the case of Hurricane Katrina. The aftereffects may include the following:

- Temporary or permanent out-migration of the population (After hurricanes Katrina and Rita, many New Orleans and Gulf Coast residents moved out of the area.)
- Temporary or permanent out-migration of physicians, nurses, other caregivers, management, and line staff (Hurricane Katrina destroyed housing on the Gulf Coast, where many hospital employees and clinicians lived. Hospitals in the area sustained a shortage of nurses and physicians, many of whom started new practices elsewhere and do not plan to return.)
- Temporary or permanent in-migration of population (An influx of new residents may require new and more services, more staff, re-analysis of community needs, and review of already established plans.)
- Increase in the uninsured and underinsured
- Increase in local wages and recruitment and retention challenges (Involvement in recovery efforts in the area—such as cleanup, disaster management, and new construction—may take workers away from their hospital jobs.)
- Need for employee financial assistance and counseling
- Impairment of employee morale
- New and lost business opportunities (Disasters may damage existing service lines, but they may also usher in new opportunities, such as behavioral health, employee assistance programs, and rehabilitation services.)

Here are some questions for evaluating whether the organization can handle a long-term impairment of its revenue stream:

- How can the current payment policy and collection process be followed in a damaged economy? Are changes needed now?
- Where will financing for impaired operations come from?
- How will personnel shortages and consequent recruitment be financed?
- How does the loss of revenue affect the organization's relationship with vendors, banks, and bondholders?
- Does the organization have the capability or relationships to seek special assistance from local, state, and federal governments?

Considering the effects of possible outcomes during catastrophe financial planning allows the organization to structure a plan that is comprehensive, realistic, and proactive rather than reactive.

CONCLUSION

In financial or risk management planning for catastrophic events, the hospital should place as much emphasis on disaster preparedness as on recovery. The CFO plays a critical role in this planning and should be an advocate or a leader in this effort. The chief executive officer should follow up with those responsible for planning to ensure that plans are developed according to identified needs. Chapter 7 continues this financial planning discussion, focusing on what the financial team should do during and after a disaster.

Financial Actions During and After the Catastrophe

Chapter 6 discussed the importance of financially preparing the healthcare organization for a catastrophe and the elements to consider and include for that type of planning. While that chapter focused on the activities before a disaster hits, this chapter addresses the specific actions to take during and after the event. These activities (Exhibit 7.1) follow the framework laid out in Chapter 6:

◆ Apply for payer advances, if needed.
◆ Exercise the line of credit.
◆ Organize information for filing insurance and FEMA (Federal Emergency Management Agency) claims.
◆ File insurance claim.
◆ Apply for FEMA reimbursement and grants.
◆ Work with the bond trustee and credit enhancement firm.
◆ Locate other funding sources.

Each of these actions is discussed in the sections that follow.

Exhibit 7.1 Checklist for Financial Actions During and After a Catastrophe

- Apply for payer advances, if needed.
- Exercise the line of credit.
- Organize information for filing insurance and FEMA (Federal Emergency Management Agency) claims.
- File insurance claim.
- Apply for FEMA reimbursement and grants.
- Work with the bond trustee and credit enhancement firm.
- Locate other funding sources.

APPLY FOR PAYER ADVANCES

An organization's good relationship with its major payers may enable it to seek an advance from payers when the organization's billing operations are disrupted or if the payer's normal claims-paying operations are disrupted. Medicare, for example, can make provisions for emergency payment advances in certain situations. Arrange these advances through the organization's fiscal intermediary. Specific rules apply regarding the timing of repayment. Negotiate and lay out the circumstances for and terms of an advance in the managed care contracts before an emergency occurs.

Keep in mind that the payer may worry that the hospital will not be able to resume operations and repay the advance. However, requesting a normal incurred-but-not-reported (IBNR) advance from payers is reasonable; that is, the organization may submit an estimate of the IBNR claims for each payer's patients at any given time. This estimate may include DNFB (discharged but not final billed) accounts, in-house charges, and other bills in accounts receivable. An IBNR advance agreement should follow a formula—for example, 30 days' advance of normal activity by the payer is to be repaid 25 percent per month, beginning 90 days after receiving the advance.

EXERCISE THE LINE OF CREDIT

The line of credit the organization has obtained (see Chapter 6) is a dependable source of funds during a disaster. Immediately after normal operations are disrupted, you may not know exactly the extent and consequences of the damage and if the line of credit will be used (or how much of it, for that matter). But even if you do not think the line of credit needs to be tapped, you should draw a small amount to understand and test the required approval processes and the time frame involved for such a transaction. Exercising the line of credit not only gives the organization some cash to use but also prepares the organization and the bank for future draws—during the recovery phase, for example.

ORGANIZE INFORMATION FOR FILING INSURANCE AND FEMA CLAIMS

Filing insurance and FEMA claims is a detailed, multistep initiative. Preparing to file is as important as the filing itself. As mentioned in Chapter

6, the first steps in this effort are to form a claims-filing team and provide training. This section covers the processes beyond the initial steps. A critical note is in order at this point: The claims team must not engage in premature or unofficial communication with the insurance company or FEMA because such exchanges could damage the claim. All communications must be kept at a professional and cordial level and should flow only from designated team members.

Information Collection

Set up an area that can be used by the team for claims-related activity, including information collection (see Exhibit 7.2 for a list of items needed). This area should be equipped with a filing system for the data and documents collected; each identified item of loss should have its own folder. Put a dedicated scanner and copier in this area to make electronic files of the documents. Having a full electronic version of your claim will prove invaluable later.

During planning, create a form—preferably the HICS (hospital incident command system) form or something comparable to it—that can be used for reporting damage or business interruption. Ideally, this form is filled out electronically, but a paper form is certainly workable and can be easily attached as a cover sheet to

---

Exhibit 7.2 Checklist of the Documents Needed for Filing a Claim

- Insurance policy
- Fixed-asset list
- Audited financial statements for the last five years
- Departmental performance reports (budget versus actual)
- Medicare cost reports for the last five years
- Invoices at time of purchase of damaged equipment
- Log of disaster timeline, including time (start and end) of damage or business interruption
- Digital pictures of each damaged item (before and after repair)
- List of actions taken to minimize damage or business interruption
- Completed forms (e.g., HICS) that document damage or business interruption
- Tracking system for each item damaged or for business interruption
- Invoices or estimates for repairs
- Quotes for replacements

---

other documents. This form must be completed immediately at the beginning of the disaster.

Establish a tracking system for each item damaged or for business interruption. This system could be as simple as assigning each item a number, which can be linked to the folder that contains all the information for that item. The numbers may be stored in an Excel database and should be kept secure, with access to the information limited only to authorized personnel.

Accounting for business interruption loss is special. By definition, business interruption does not get reported in the regular accounting system. Business does not come in, so no income is reported. Therefore, each department should record what activities are *not* happening so that the claims team and forensic accountants can accurately estimate the lost income.

Take digital pictures of each item that sustained damage immediately after the damage occurs. If the damage must be repaired (to prevent further damage, for example) before the adjuster arrives, before-and-after pictures of the item will document the loss. These pictures should be printed and put in their respective folders, and backup and electronic copies should be saved. Name each set of pictures clearly—for example, the department name, item name, and date taken could be used as the filename. Even if the camera is set to include the date and time stamp on the printed pictures, you should add the date to the filename. This detailed naming convention helps the claims team easily and quickly identify the files needed.

Cleanup and Debris Removal

Catastrophes often cause damages, such as downed trees, that obstruct access to the facility. In this case, the best action to take is to get and document several quotes for debris removal and select the best, immediate service. The goal here is to show that the organization took the reasonable step to clear debris and clean up the campus to mitigate the business interruption and to continue operations, while also having obtained competitive quotes. Then, the organization can later file a claim with the insurance company and FEMA.

FEMA pays to have downed trees removed if they are within 200 feet of a structure, but check current regulations to ensure what service will be reimbursed. And consider that these removal contracts take weeks or even months for FEMA to arrange. Waiting is not a good option, especially because rubble, debris, or other obstructions give the public the idea that the organization is closed for business.

FILE INSURANCE CLAIM

As listed in Exhibit 7.3, immediately after a catastrophe hits, the organization must notify the insurance broker and carrier so that they can arrange for the designated adjuster to inspect the damage as soon as possible.

Insurance carriers require that the proper process for filing a claim is followed. But the most important element of filing is the documentation that must accompany the claim. The documentation must be thorough, providing clear support for the claim.

For example, if certain equipment was damaged because the disaster cut off power that, in turn, made the room in which the equipment was stored too hot, the insurance carrier will require the facility to show that the staff (1) took proper actions to keep the equipment from failing, such as moving it to a cooler area, and (2) performed maintenance and calibration at the right time. In other words, the documentation must prove that the

---

Exhibit 7.3 Checklist for Filing a Claim (Post-Loss)

- Contact the insurance broker and carrier immediately. In the case of a predictable catastrophe, such as a hurricane headed for the area within 48 hours, put the broker, carrier, adjuster, and other involved parties on notice. Demand on the carrier (not to mention the adjusters) will be heavy during and after the storm. By acting sooner, your claim will be set in motion before the catastrophe occurs. If a pre-loss meeting is conducted, the adjuster already has all the pertinent information about the policy.

- Bring the claims team together with other parties, such as the broker, independent accountants, and engineers, to assist in the claims process.

- Follow the established claims process and the designated target dates and action items until the claim is closed.

- Keep a disaster log to document times, places, and any information related to the catastrophe and consequent damage or business interruption. This documentation is part of the insurance paperwork.

- Build an internal database of the damages. This database serves as the general repository of the documentation maintained, such as the disaster log. The accounting department should be assigned to update the database as more information comes in.

- Conduct an internal assessment of the damages. Personnel at the hospital may be most qualified to perform this assessment because they are physically at the site.

- Conduct a meeting with the adjuster to review and assess the damages.

- Process a request for an advance (the amount of which is based on the assessed damages), with a target of 30 days from the date of loss or business interruption.

- Motivate the claims team to move the process along to closure and to ensure that the recovery is in line with the loss and insurance policy provisions.

---

damage was caused by the disaster, not by improper handling or normal wear and tear. If the documentation is incomplete or questionable, the claim payment will be delayed at best and denied at worst—a situation that can lead to lengthy negotiations and even costly litigation. If the documentation proves that the equipment was indeed damaged by the catastrophe, the organization should insist on replacement rather than repairs because repaired equipment tends to pose patient-safety risks. However, replacing equipment, especially if an upgrade is required, could cause the hospital to exceed its certificate-of-need (CON) expenditure threshold. During the planning stage, the team should check CON rules with a CON agency and obtain the requirements in writing.

Documentation for damage and business interruption of a sizable scope usually takes up several thick notebooks. For business interruption, the documentation includes the financial statements, cost reports, and analytical spreadsheets that detail loss of income prepared by the claims team and forensic accountants. This information should demonstrate the following:

◆ *The period (start and end) of business interruption.* This time frame should comply with the definition stated in the insurance policy.

◆ *The impact on operations during the period of interruption.* Cases, days, procedures, and revenues should be included for the prior three to five years during the same month(s) that the interruption occurred, not the months in the interrupted period. For example, if the interruption happened in June, July, and August, volume and revenue data should be provided for June, July, and August in the past three to five years, not the data for June, July, and August in the current year.

◆ *The expenses incurred during the period of interruption.* Knowing what the policy covers enables the claims team to advise the CEO and other administrators on what expenses to continue or cut in the aftermath of a disaster. For example, critical nursing, professional staff, and support staff must be retained, but their activities must involve those that minimize losses, even if these activities differ from what they normally do. During an interruption, asking staff to clean and sanitize equipment, supplies, and patient care units; transfer to other departments with the most need; or develop and implement new policies and procedures is reasonable.

◆ *The projected increase in business during the period of interruption.* Be realistic about this part of the claim. The documentation should prove that the organization was projected to increase income in the period the disaster occurred, but unrealistic projections could delay payment or generate possible accusations of fraud or abuse. Even if the business was on a recent uptick, the insurer may not be convinced that the increase would have happened during the period. Good documentation of the loss and the projections prevents doubts and questions and helps to bring the claim a fair consideration.

In any claims, conflict between the insured and the carrier is likely. But conflict can be minimized with solid preparation before the need arises and good documentation during and after the event.

APPLY FOR FEMA REIMBURSEMENT AND GRANTS

FEMA's website (www.fema.org) contains information on its rules and regulations. This website is invaluable to planners, as it lays out what FEMA covers, what reimbursements and grants it offers, how to file claims, and so on. Exhibit 7.4 is a reprint of FEMA's "Disaster Assistance Policy 9525.4: Emergency Medical Care and Medical Evacuations." This guideline discusses how healthcare facilities can obtain assistance from FEMA. Check the FEMA website for updates to this policy.

Exhibit 7.4 Emergency Medical Care and Medical Evacuations

Disaster Assistance Policy 9525.4

- **TITLE:** Emergency Medical Care and Medical Evacuations
- **DATE:** July 16, 2008
- **PURPOSE:**

This policy identifies the extraordinary emergency medical care and medical evacuation expenses that are eligible for reimbursement under the *Category B, Emergency Protective Measures* provision of the Federal Emergency Management Agency's (FEMA) Public Assistance Program following an emergency or major disaster declaration.

- **SCOPE AND AUDIENCE:**

The policy is applicable to all emergencies and major disasters declared on or after the date of publication of this policy. It is intended for FEMA and State personnel involved in the administration of the Public Assistance Program.

- **AUTHORITY:**

Sections 403 and 502 of the Robert T. Stafford Disaster Relief and Emergency Assistance Act (Stafford Act), 42 U.S.C. §§ 5170b and 5192, respectively, and Title 44 of the Code of Federal Regulations (CFR)§ 206.225

- **BACKGROUND:**

- Sections 403 and 502 of the Stafford Act authorize Federal agencies to provide assistance, including emergency medical care, essential to meeting immediate threats to life and property resulting from a major disaster or emergency, respectively. When the emergency medical delivery system within the designated disaster area is destroyed or severely compromised by a disaster event, assistance for emergency medical care and medical evacuations of disaster victims from eligible public and private nonprofit hospitals and custodial care facilities is available to eligible Public Assistance applicants through Public Assistance grants, Direct Federal Assistance (DFA), or a combination of both.

- When the State and local governments lack the capability to perform or contract for eligible emergency medical care or medical evacuation work, they may request Direct Federal Assistance from FEMA. Usually, FEMA will task the appropriate Federal agencies via mission assignments to perform the requested emergency work. FEMA may task the Department of Health and Human Services to provide emergency medical assistance when requested by the State.

(continued)

Exhibit 7.4 Emergency Medical Care and Medical Evacuations (continued)

Disaster Assistance Policy 9525.4 (continued)

- **POLICY:**
  - **Definitions**
    - Cost-to-charge ratio: A ratio established by Medicare to estimate a medical service provider's actual costs in relation to its charges
    - Durable medical equipment: Equipment prescribed by a physician that is medically necessary for the treatment of an illness or injury, or to prevent a patient's further deterioration. This equipment is designed for repeated use and includes items such as oxygen equipment, wheelchairs, walkers, hospital beds, crutches, and other medical equipment.
    - Emergency Management Assistance Compact: A mutual aid agreement and partnership between states in which disaster-impacted states can request and receive reimbursable assistance from other member states
    - Emergency medical care: Medical treatment or services provided for injuries, illnesses, and conditions caused as a direct result of the emergency or declared disaster, and which require immediate medical treatment or services to evaluate and stabilize an emergency medical condition. Emergency medical care may include care provided during transport under a medical evacuation and stabilization of persons injured during evacuation.
    - Operating costs: Costs of personnel, equipment, and supplies required to operate a facility, and costs of the facility itself
  - **Eligible Applicants.** Eligible applicants may include State and local governments and private nonprofit organizations or institutions that own or operate a medical or custodial care facility, such as a publicly owned or private nonprofit hospital or nursing home (44 CFR 206.221, and 206.222). Private for-profit medical service providers are not eligible applicants for Public Assistance. However, some costs associated with for-profit providers may be eligible for Public Assistance when contracted for by an eligible applicant.
  - **Eligible Emergency Medical Care Costs.** Eligible applicants may be eligible to receive Public Assistance funding for the extraordinary costs associated with providing temporary facilities for emergency medical care of disaster victims when existing facilities are overwhelmed. Costs associated with emergency medical care should be reasonable and customary for the emergency medical services provided. Where applicable, FEMA may rely on Medicare's cost-to-charge ratio to determine the reasonableness of costs. Eligible costs will be limited to a period of up to 30 days from the date of the emergency or disaster declaration, or as determined by the Federal Coordinating Officer.
    - Eligible costs include, but are not limited to, the following:
      - Overtime for regular full-time employees performing eligible work
      - Regular time and overtime for extra hires specifically hired to provide additional support as a result of the emergency or declared disaster (*see* FEMA Recovery Policy RP9525.7, *Labor Costs–Emergency Work*, for information related to eligible labor costs while performing emergency work)
      - Transport of disaster victims requiring emergency medical care to medical facilities, including EMS and ambulance services

- **Eligible Emergency Medical Care Costs** *(continued)*.
  - Treatment and monitoring of disaster victims requiring emergency medical care, including costs for:
    - Triage, medically necessary testing, and diagnosis
    - First-aid assessment and provision of first aid, including materials (bandages, etc.)
    - Prescription assistance limited to a one-time 30-day supply for acute conditions and to replace maintenance prescriptions
    - Durable medical equipment
  - Vaccinations for disaster victims and emergency workers, including medical staff
  - Provision of health information
  - Temporary tents or portable buildings for treatment of disaster victims
  - Leased or purchased equipment for use in temporary facilities (*see* FEMA Recovery Policy RP9523.3, *Provision of Temporary Relocation Facilities,* for information related to the eligibility of costs associated with leasing and purchasing temporary facilities)
  - Security for temporary facilities
  - Ineligible costs include the following:
  - Medical care costs incurred once a disaster victim is admitted to a medical care facility on an inpatient basis
  - Costs associated with follow-on treatment of disaster victims beyond 30 days of the emergency or disaster declaration
  - Increased administrative and operating costs to the hospital due to increased or anticipated increased patient load
  - Loss of revenue
  - Ineligible costs remain ineligible even if incurred under mutual aid or other assistance agreements.
  - Eligible costs of emergency medical care provided in congregate or transitional shelters are addressed in FEMA Disaster Assistance Policy DAP9523.15, *Eligible Costs Related to Evacuations and Sheltering.*

- **Eligible Medical Evacuation Costs.** Disasters can so seriously threaten or cause such severe damage to eligible medical and custodial facilities that patients have to be evacuated and transported to either a temporary facility or to an existing facility that has spare capacity. When an evacuation is required, there may be eligible costs incurred by an eligible applicant in the evacuation and transportation of patients, such as the use of emergency medical service personnel or ambulance services.
  - Eligible costs include, but are not limited to, the following:
    - Overtime for regular full-time employees to evacuate and assist in the transport of patients from the original facility

(continued)

Exhibit 7.4 Emergency Medical Care and Medical Evacuations (continued)

- Regular time and overtime of extra hires employed to evacuate and assist in the transport of patients from the original facility (*see* FEMA Recovery Policy RP9525.7, *Labor Costs–Emergency Work,* for information related to eligible labor costs while performing emergency work)

- Equipment costs incurred in the transport of patients from the original facility

- Labor and equipment costs incurred during transport while returning the patient to the original medical or custodial care facility

- The costs of treatment of patients requiring emergency medical care, including costs for medically necessary tests, medication, and durable medical equipment required to stabilize patients for transportation

- Costs incurred from the activation of contracts, mutual aid agreements, or force account resources in advance of an emergency or disaster event necessary to prepare for medical evacuations in threatened areas. Eligible equipment costs include mobilization of ambulances and other transport equipment; eligible force account labor costs are limited to overtime for regular full-time employees and regular time and overtime of extra hires.

- Ineligible costs include equipment and labor costs incurred during standby times.

- **Duplication of Benefits.** FEMA is prohibited by Section 312 of the Stafford Act from approving funds for reimbursement that are covered by any other source of funding. Therefore, eligible applicants must take reasonable steps to prevent such an occurrence and provide documentation on a patient-by-patient basis verifying that insurance coverage or any other source of funding—including private insurance, Medicaid, or Medicare—has been pursued and does not exist for the costs associated with emergency medical care and emergency medical evacuations.

- **Preparation Costs.** Costs incurred in preparation for an increased patient load from an emergency or disaster, including costs of personnel, emergency medical equipment, and standby for ambulance services and emergency medical service personnel, are not eligible for Public Assistance grant funding.

- **Mutual Aid.** The Emergency Management Assistance Compact (EMAC) between states and other individual mutual aid agreements can be used to provide emergency medical care in an emergency or major disaster. Costs incurred through these mutual aid agreements may be eligible for Public Assistance grant funding. Reimbursement claims made by mutual aid providers must comply with the requirements of FEMA Disaster Assistance Policy DAP9523.6, *Mutual Aid Agreements for Public Assistance and Fire Management Assistance.* Public or private nonprofit medical service providers working within their jurisdiction do not qualify as mutual aid providers under DAP9523.6.

- **RESPONSIBLE OFFICE:** Disaster Assistance Directorate (Public Assistance Division)

As is done for insurance claims, applying for FEMA grants and reimbursements requires the team to be organized and methodical. Filing systems and spreadsheets help with recordkeeping, activity tracking, costs incurred, damage sustained, and change (e.g., hiring) in personnel needs and spending. Careful documentation enables the organization to quickly take appropriate advantage of FEMA funds.

The team should review each FEMA-eligible item in Exhibit 7.4 and document the incurrence of the item and its cost. The tracking methods for FEMA are the same as for insurance claims filing. FEMA payment typically takes longer than insurance payment, because FEMA will not pay for something that is covered by insurance.

Most important, an organization that is aware of the available FEMA reimbursements and grants can make better operational decisions in the aftermath of a disaster. For example, under FEMA's emergency-care reimbursement policy, a facility can hire more staff, pay overtime for existing staff, set up tents and portable sections for triage and treatment, offer prescription assistance, transport patients, and much more. A facility that does not know about such funding may be restrained in providing such services and assistance to the community.

WORK WITH THE BOND TRUSTEE AND CREDIT ENHANCEMENT FIRM

If a healthcare organization has issued bonds, a "bond trustee" acts on behalf of the bondholders. Often, but not always, the healthcare organization improves the interest rate by engaging a "credit enhancement firm" such as a bond insurer or bank. The credit enhancement firm guarantees payment of the debt to the bondholders in case of default by the healthcare organization.

A hospital's bond issue includes definitions for circumstances that require trustee approval or authorization, such as damage repair. For example, the bond document may have a damage threshold of 10 percent of book value; if damage is greater than that, the healthcare organization has to get authorization from the bond trustee before making repairs. This provision protects the bondholders, who may prefer to take the insurance money than use it to repair equipment that may not be worth repairing. For example, if the damage is significant (say, 60 percent or above) and the surrounding population is diminished, the healthcare organization's future financial performance may be suspect, so the bondholders might take the insurance money rather than repair the equipment. In some cases, this situation could result in the facility closing permanently or reopening only under new ownership and capitalization. This situation happened in New Orleans, where the post-Katrina population declined significantly and some hospitals just stayed closed. Exhibit 7.5 lists the steps for dealing with the bond trustee.

In any communication with the bond trustee and credit enhancement firm, the organization's representative should project knowledge and confidence about the actions being taken by the institution. This will engender trust between the trustee and the organization and put the trustee's mind at ease that the organization is in full control of the situation at hand.

Exhibit 7.5 Steps for Dealing with the Bond Trustee

- Understand the organization's bond covenants and create a flowchart of the decision tree.
- Contact the bond trustee and credit enhancement firm immediately after the disaster, and establish a contact person with the firm.
- Prepare a written update for the trustee and credit enhancement firm within the first week after the disaster. This update should include the following information:
  - Insurance coverage
  - Expected amount of insurance and FEMA claims
  - Status of business interruption and resumption
- Review the update weekly by conference call until things stabilize, the claim is paid, and the annual audit is complete.

LOCATE OTHER FUNDING SOURCES

Following are ways to seek additional funding:

- Contact the office of the governor to formally request a federal disaster declaration for the affected area. Such a declaration will open up opportunities for special funding and incentives, including FEMA assistance. The state's emergency management agency can provide this information.
- Contact your area's congressional representatives.
- Partner with other hospitals and providers in the area to leverage their relationships with governmental offices and to structure a special assistance request.

CONCLUSION

Creating a solid financial plan and implementing it swiftly following a catastrophe are critical to the long-term stability of the facility. Take the strategies discussed in Chapter 6 to develop an initial framework for disaster financial planning. Then, during and after the disaster, apply the ideas discussed in this chapter. Last, encourage the staff to devote time to planning, as that will greatly mitigate the damage and interruption that a catastrophic event can bring.

CHAPTER 8

What's in Our Future?

Loss of life and property; permanent and temporary disruptions; and financial, emotional, physical, and mental tolls are just some of the myriad outcomes of a catastrophe. Preparations for disasters are absolutely necessary, and so is awareness of the natural and man-made dangers in the world. Some of these threats may be predicted to minimize (if not prevent) damages and loss, while others are unforeseeable and random. In any event, individuals, healthcare administrators and organizations, and communities must educate themselves about these risks so that they can protect themselves and perhaps even participate in efforts to ward off disasters.

This chapter discusses the existing conditions in the world that could culminate in a catastrophe in the near or distant future. These threats—products of both environmental and man-made factors—are often interrelated and challenge our current views and practices.

CLIMATE AND TEMPERATURE CHANGE

If you casually observe the weather in the United States alone, you will notice unusual weather events: Perhaps Oregon experienced a warm winter, while Louisiana saw some snow. Although these instances are not enough to declare that global warming is the cause, they do indicate that changes are coming (*Digital Journal* 2010). More heat waves seem to be occurring in big cities, such as Atlanta, Houston, Chicago, and New York. According to "an analysis of weather records at Georgia Tech...the average number of heat-wave days in large U.S. cities each year had increased from 9 in the mid-1950s to 19 by the mid-2000s" (Stone 2010). Furthermore, the National Climatic Data Center, which has been keeping temperature records since 1880, found that 2005 was the warmest year, but 2010 could take this distinction (msnbc.com 2010).

These observations also apply to the rest of the world. Consider the following findings:

- Global surface temperatures in 2009, according to provisional World Meteorological Organization data, were 0.44 degrees Celsius above the 1961–1990 average of 14 degrees celsius. The decade of 2000 to 2009 was the warmest since 1850 (Faust 2009).
- In 2005, the Intergovernmental Panel on Climate Change (IPCC) and the Arctic Climate Impact Assessment found that warming was progressing much faster in the Arctic regions than predicted in even the worst-case scenario laid out in the 2001 IPCC report (UNEP 2006).
- In the 20th century, the global climate heated 0.74 degrees Celsius, with the 10 hottest years on record having occurred within the recent past (Glantz and Ye 2010, 57).
- Heat waves are major killers and may become a greater health threat in the 21st century, especially in urban areas (Glantz and Ye 2010).

Scientists use computer models to generate scenarios brought on by a warmer atmosphere, including the following (Associated Press 2005):

- More intense (Category 5) and frequent storms, including hurricanes, typhoons, and cyclones
- More droughts, floods, and fires
- A poleward movement (expanding to the north and south poles) of tropical diseases
- Global changes in the expected flow of the seasons

Climate change inevitably has considerable effects on people's health and, by extension, healthcare organizations. The Interagency Working Group on Climate Change and Health (2008) developed a white paper to call attention to this issue. The group contends that climate change may bring about, or possibly exacerbate, the following health hazards:

- Asthma, respiratory allergies, and airway diseases
- Cancer
- Cardiovascular disease and stroke
- Food-borne diseases
- Heat-related morbidity and mortality
- Human developmental problems
- Mental health and stress-related disorders

- Neurological diseases and disorders
- Vector-borne (through ticks, mosquitoes, and rodents) and zoonotic (from animal to human) diseases
- Waterborne diseases
- Weather-related morbidity and mortality

For healthcare organizations, climate change could mean "resource scarcity and the possibility of transportation and other social system (electricity, communications, manufacturing, water and sewer) breakdowns or interruptions. Specific to the medical care system, electronic medical records as well as radiology, laboratory, and a host of other medical services, which depend upon an uninterrupted power source and low energy costs, will be at risk" (Bednarz and Bradford 2008).

As Glantz and Ye (2010, 224–25) argue, improving how we deal with climate extremes today can help us cope with them in the future.

SEA-LEVEL RISE AND ICE MELT

The National Wetlands Research Center defines sea-level rise as the "rise in the surface of the sea due to increased water volume of the ocean and/or sinking of the land." This phenomenon is linked to global warming, wind patterns, ocean currents, and even land collapse, which may explain why the increase in sea levels is different from one region to the next (Lemonick 2010). Low-lying areas, small islands, and deltas are vulnerable to sea-level increase, and news that this level is rising faster than predicted is sobering. The current estimate is that by 2100, the sea level will rise about a meter (Lemonick 2010).

Melting polar ice is a contributor to sea-level rise, although some observers contend that this contribution is not significant. However, consider the following reports:

- "The loss of that [Antarctic] ice sheet alone would inundate some coastal areas, swamping New York, Washington DC, south Florida, Los Angeles, San Francisco, and Seattle, with sea levels in some places higher by 21 feet or more" (Dunham 2009).
- "Sea ice cover is currently decreasing by 11.2 percent per decade relative to the 1979–2000 average, and thinning of the ice in winter is especially significant. Thus, the volume of ice has fallen significantly" (Munich Re 2009).
- In recent years, the sea ice has reduced during the Arctic winter from around 3 meters to 2.4 meters, the trend being an annual decrease of 0.17 meters (Kwok et al. 2009, Kwok and Rothrock 2009 in Munich Re 2009).

- "Over the period of modern satellite observations (1979-present) Arctic sea ice extent at the end of the melt season has declined at a rate of more than 11 percent per decade, and there is evidence that the rate of decline has accelerated during the last decade. According to Kwok et al (2009) the Arctic Ocean has lost 40 percent of its multiyear ice in the last five years" (Kattsov et al. 2010; Kwok and Rothrock 2009).
- "By the end of this century, Arctic readings could rise to levels not seen in 130,000 years. Even now, giant glaciers lubricated by melting water have begun causing earthquakes in Greenland as they lurch toward the ocean" (Schmid 2006).
- "Ice sheets have melted before and sea levels rose. The warmth needed isn't that much above present conditions" (Schmid 2006).

The 2007 report "Nation Under Siege," by The 2030 Research Center, addresses the impact of rising sea level on the coastal towns and cities of the United States, including San Francisco, San Diego, Seattle, Boston, New York, and Miami. The report includes illustrations that depict how these areas, their infrastructures, and their populace will be inundated by rising water. In addition, the report discusses those who may be hit hardest if these scenarios occurred, such as people who do not have a vehicle, do not speak English, or live near hazardous waste facilities. Low-income households and communities of color make up the bulk of these vulnerable groups. See the report at http://solveclimate.com/resource/nation-under-siege.

WATER SHORTAGE

The world is 80 percent water, an irony in the face of water shortage. Some estimates say that only 1 percent of the world's water is drinkable, as the rest is salty sea water (97 percent) and water in polar ice (2 percent). Overpopulation, pollution, poor water management, agricultural and industry booms, urbanization, and climate change are just some of the causes of water shortage.

A recent study sponsored by the National Resources Defense Council (2010) found that 1,100 counties in the continental United States are at high risk for a water shortage by 2050. These areas are located in Arizona, Arkansas, California, Colorado, Florida, Idaho, Kansas, Mississippi, Montana, Nebraska, Nevada, New Mexico, Oklahoma, and Texas. Worldwide, the facts are bleaker: "The World Health Organization says more than one billion people live in areas where renewable water resources are not available. The problem is especially serious in Asia and the Pacific...[where] nearly seven hundred thousand people...lack safe drinking water" (VOA News.com 2010). This combined area is second only to the African continent, where water shortage is dire.

The consequences of the lack or inadequate supply of water are not hard to imagine. Following are the unfortunate realities in hospitals in water-deprived countries:

- In Kenya, "hospitals, like Kakamega Provincial District General Hospital, where Hellen Wasiliwa has recently given birth, are often forced to collect rain water in buckets to meet the needs of their patients. Due to severe shortages, the limited water supply is usually shared among patients and is also most often not purified or disinfected" (Njeru 2010).
- In Nepal, "Patients in the district hospital have been hit hard due to the acute shortage of water. They were compelled to buy water from shops or relatives of patients…fetch[ed] water for them due to the lack of water in the hospital" (*The Himalayan Times* 2010).
- In Turkey, "due to the water shortage, some hospitals stopped admitting patients except for urgent cases, while some delayed non-vital surgical operations. Moreover, the water shortage increased the risk of disease" (Ikinci 2007).

Death, spread and multiplication of disease, poor sanitation, and inability to provide a basic necessity are just some of the grave consequences of the water crisis. Preparing for this threat is not just a healthcare duty but a world mandate.

TERRORISM AND BIOTERRORISM

Since September 11, 2001, Americans have been on high alert for the next wave of terrorism (internal and external) that could hit us on a grand scale. And since September 11 alone, several minor attacks and threats have occurred on U.S. soil. Fortunately, such threats have been foiled. But still, the threat of another terrorist attack, including bioterrorism, is real.

Earlier in 2010, a congressional hearing on the National Strategy for Countering Biological Threats was held, in which "the acting assistant secretary of State for the Bureau of International Security and Nonproliferation, testified that 'The biological threat has several important components, including intent from groups that have expressed interest in obtaining biological weapons and expertise, emerging infectious diseases that create new opportunities for havoc, and growing biotechnology capacity in areas of the world with a terrorist presence…. A biological weapons attack is a real and present danger, particularly in light of the 2001 anthrax attacks'" (Kraft 2010).

Bioterrorism—the use of biological agents (germs, bacteria, and viruses) to imperil, injure, or kill people, animals, and even plant life—is bolstered by the availability of the necessary harmful agents as well as the fast spread and severity of illness or disease. The Centers for Disease Control and Prevention (CDC) has created a comprehensive web page dedicated to bioterrorism. This page includes a list of biological agents; facts about each agent such as its health effects; information for first responders in an event of a biological attack; and preparation and planning recommendations for healthcare facilities. See http://emergency.cdc.gov/bioterrorism.

PANDEMIC INFLUENZA AND EMERGING INFECTIOUS DISEASES

A pandemic is a global outbreak of disease. In June 2009, the World Health Organization (WHO) declared the H1N1 influenza (swine flu) a pandemic, after two months filled with confirmed cases (and deaths) in North America, Mexico, and Europe. Fear of contracting, spreading, and dying from the virus was high, and the world's governments and health departments were on high alert, issuing public information and cautionary announcements and ordering big batches of vaccines. Fortunately, the projected death tolls did not materialize. Unfortunately, the overall hype and media coverage of the H1N1 events turned off many people—some doubted the vaccine's safety, while some questioned WHO's motivation to declare the outbreak a pandemic, claiming the organization was influenced by pharmaceutical companies. As a result, 40 million doses of the vaccine went unused and have been thrown away (Gupta 2010). Make no mistake, however: H1N1 is still an active health threat. WHO still urges health departments and individuals to be vigilant. In addition, the United Nations posts weekly updates and news about H1N1 from across the world on its website. See www.un-influenza.org.

Another real threat is the avian flu (H5N1 virus). The avian flu is an infection in birds (e.g., chickens, ducks, geese) that can be transferred to humans through direct or close contact with the contaminated bird (dead or alive). Cases of the H5N1 in humans have been reported in Asia, Africa, and Europe; there have been 502 laboratory-confirmed cases, of whom 298 died (Kaiser Family Foundation 2010). Recent H5N1 deaths or new cases have been reported in Indonesia, Vietnam, Nepal, Egypt, Singapore, China, and Myanmar; cases have also been reported in Europe. In the United States, according to the CDC (n.d.), "Highly pathogenic avian influenza A (H5N1) viruses have never been detected among wild birds, domestic poultry, or people in the United States." For more and up-to-date information on the avian flu, visit the websites of WHO (www.who.int/csr/disease/avian_influenza/en) and the CDC (www.cdc.gov/flu/avian/gen-info/qa.htm).

Some highly contagious illnesses that occurred in the past (often as an epidemic) are now coming back for another round of attacks on humans. Examples of these diseases include West Nile virus, SARS (severe acute respiratory syndrome), *E. coli*, anthrax, tuberculosis, malaria, lyme disease, small pox, dengue fever, and AIDS. According to the National Institute of Allergy and Infectious Diseases (n.d.), "despite remarkable advances in medical research and treatments during the 20th century, infectious diseases remain among the leading causes of death worldwide." The latest alerts and announcements about emerging diseases can be found on *Infectious Disease News* at www.infectiousdiseasenews.com.

CONCLUSION

The publication *Planet in Peril* (UNEP 2006) named the following threats to our future:

◆ Polar ice caps melting faster
◆ Global warming
◆ Water becoming a rarity
◆ Ocean resources under threat
◆ Nuclear power for civilian and military use
◆ Weapons of mass destruction
◆ Hunger
◆ Genetically modified organisms and the threat to food crops
◆ Urban development trends
◆ Widening healthcare gap

A lot of progress is being made in minimizing the effects of these problems or eliminating them altogether, from grassroots efforts to international collaboratives. But much work needs to be done, and that work can be endless. The most practical actions in this time of environmental and man-made threats are to be correctly informed, to be vigilant, and to be prepared for all types of consequences. Those actions work for individuals, institutions, businesses, governments—for everyone. And for healthcare executives, it is imperative to remember that there are no disasters or catastrophic events that do not impact the healthcare delivery system. It is crucial that we stop debating whether the scientists are correct, and begin preparing with great vigilance.

Part IV

LESSONS LEARNED: FRONTLINE INTERVIEWS

A New Era of Terrorism: JFK Medical Center and the First Anthrax Exposure

Interview with Phillip D. Robinson, former chief executive officer, JFK Medical Center, Atlantis, Florida

Three weeks after the September 11, 2001, attacks, a patient arrived at the JFK Medical Center emergency department exhibiting symptoms of fever and delirium. An initial examination resulted in a tentative diagnosis of meningitis, but the spinal tap that followed revealed that the patient had been exposed to anthrax. Phil Robinson, CEO of JFK Medical Center at the time, restored order to the chaos, quelled fear and questioning, and organized the recovery effort. Below he describes his experience.

Interviewer: Please describe what happened during this experience.

Phillip D. Robinson (PDR): A patient was admitted to the hospital with anthrax. This was just a few weeks after 9/11 so the suspicion was that this could be the next wave of terrorist attacks. Given the climate at the time, this event generated worldwide attention, and we were swept into a situation that involved everyone from the CDC to the FBI, the Joint Chiefs of Staff, and the White House. The media attention we were given was overwhelming.

Because the source of the exposure wasn't known, there was a lot of concern that it might have come from inside the facility. At first, a lot of misinformation was circulated about anthrax and how it was contracted. We had to consider the safety of the patients and staff that were in the hospital, the privacy of the patient and the patient's family, and managing the dissemination of information both within the hospital and to the outside world with the help of the 30-plus media trucks in our front parking lot!

Interviewer: Prior to this event, how had your facility prepared for responding to a major disaster or catastrophic event? How well do you feel your facility responded to this event?

PDR: We had conducted disaster drills as a facility and in conjunction with the county. Since we were located on the Atlantic coast, we had activated our hurricane plan several times, although always had been spared a direct hit. I am not sure that anyone at that time could have adequately prepared for a bioterrorism attack or knew much about anthrax in particular. Nonetheless, many aspects of our plan were applicable to this situation.

Interviewer: Did the ownership/corporate structure of your hospital affect your response to this event?

PDR: Yes, I think so. The hospital is owned by HCA. We were given lots of support and advice during the incident by the company, and I felt as if whatever I said I needed would be provided, especially pharmaceuticals in this instance. On the other hand, I was told not to speak to the media, and at some point that became impossible because the reporters were speculating and creating panic and the patients and employees were watching it on TV. I felt that it was best to go ahead and tell the press what we knew to the extent that we could given the sensitive nature of the situation. Once we held a news conference and began posting updates on our website and through telephone messages, the HCA corporate staff was very supportive and understanding of my decision.

Interviewer: Do you feel you had the right culture to sustain you through this disaster? If so, describe the characteristics of your culture. If not, why and how would you or how have you changed the culture for future response.

PDR: We absolutely had the right culture to sustain us during this crisis. We had worked for years to create a family-like atmosphere built on trust and respect, and that definitely paid off in this instance. As difficult as it was to stay calm and focused on our patients, the team at JFK responded perfectly and professionally. Even though we didn't know how we might be personally affected, especially in the beginning when there was a possibility of us being quarantined, the staff at the hospital was just incredible. In fact, the physician who diagnosed the case had never even seen a patient with anthrax but was able to recognize the symptoms. We also never had a problem getting the staff to stay or come in and do whatever they were asked.

After the incident, we did significantly beef up our plan for infectious agents, hazardous materials, and isolation; and we also developed a much more complete plan as to how to deal with the media and communication in future situations.

Interviewer: How did you communicate internally and externally during this disaster?

PDR: We were very visible during this incident. I, along with Chief Nursing Officer Dianne Aleman, Director of Security Bill Hancsak, and VP of Marketing Madelyn Christopher, in particular, spent a lot of time in the facility and interfacing with the county health department, the CDC, the State of Florida, the physicians involved in the case, the local and Washington-based FBI teams that were on-site, and, as mentioned, the media. We also distributed written updates to each patient and employee, including the facts about anthrax and how it is contracted and spread in order to manage the message. We posted updates for our staff and others on our website and also recorded messages on the phone system.

I had no idea that there were so many jurisdictional conflicts and rivalries between the different local, state, and federal agencies. More than once I had to get everyone in the same room to make sure that we were all on the same page. I also found that a lot of the local elected officials were getting little or no official information, so I made sure that they were also kept in the loop.

Interviewer: What was the biggest challenge to your employees and your medical staff during this disaster?

PDR: I think the unknown was the biggest challenge—where had the anthrax come from, what did it mean to our own personal safety and health, who really was in charge of the situation, and which agency and officials had jurisdiction over this entire matter? That being said, ultimately, the crisis was affecting our hospital and our patients, and we had to ensure that safety, privacy, and order were maintained. I think we were able to accomplish that beautifully.

Interviewer: What agencies, individuals, or organizations were most helpful? Did any impede your ability to respond?

PDR: I was very impressed with the local field office of the FBI, as well as the CDC. The Palm Beach County Emergency Operations Center and Health Department were also very helpful and supportive, as was the secretary of health for the state of Florida. In addition, I was impressed with the number of other hospitals, even our competitors, who called and offered support and assistance. As mentioned earlier, I got a tremendous amount of support from HCA, in particular the divisional president at the time, Chuck Hall.

One thing I also learned is that at the time there was a tremendous amount of denial at all levels. More than once, Dr. Larry Bush, who brilliantly diagnosed the case along with Dr. Norman Sudduth in pathology, was told that there was no way this case could be anthrax. I have come to find out that this kind of denial is very common at the beginning of any kind of disaster or crisis.

Jurisdictional conflicts did get in the way of our initial response, as did a lack of understanding by many as to who was actually in charge of the situation. This was before the Department of Homeland Security was established with the intent to clarify these roles.

Interviewer: What do you wish you had known before this event?

PDR: I wish I had known more about bioterrorism and the agents that are used. I also wish I had known more about jurisdiction of the various agencies during disasters and catastrophes.

Interviewer: What did you do that you feel was right?

PDR: Communicate, and get all of the agencies and officials to communicate with each other. I think we did right by the patient and the patient's family in spite of the terrible situation. When we adopted the position that whatever was said or done had to be done with our involvement and blessing, it made things go a lot more smoothly. Of course, the medical professionals that diagnosed the anthrax so quickly probably saved thousands of others from getting sick or worse.

Interviewer: What three things would you do differently? How has the hospital changed after this event?

PDR: I would have had a press conference much sooner to reassure the patients in the hospital and members of the community. I would have asked for formal and routine meetings with all of the agencies and authorities involved to make sure we all had the same information and facts. The lack of communication and competitiveness between some of these agencies was quite ridiculous, so this would be as much to help them as to help me and our hospital. Lastly, I think the hospital developed a sense of accomplishment and pride in what we had gone through and how we handled the situation. I think after this happened we were convinced we could handle almost any challenge that would be presented to us.

Of course, I have also become passionate about what leadership in a crisis means and how important it is for the CEO and others to captain the ship during these incidents.

Interviewer: What surprised or shocked you about your experience?

PDR: As I have already mentioned, the level of competition and friction between local, state, and federal agencies was something I had not encountered. The fact that the media so quickly learned of the situation even though we were under a gag order not to speak about it shows how unrealistic that position was. I think the grace under pressure that I observed in so many of the clinical and medical staff, as well as in the PR and nursing leadership, was just amazing.

Interviewer: What advice would you give for those who will face similar situations in the future?

PDR: Do not cede your authority to anyone. Be cooperative, yet force collaboration if you have to. Be visible and reassuring and remember that it is your hospital and you will be the one to get everyone back on track and focused after the incident is over.

Interviewer: What did you learn about yourself, your team, and your facility?

PDR: I don't think anything makes a team or an organization stronger than going through something like this successfully. I learned so much about the strength and character of the physicians and staff that I worked with, and also learned a lot about myself. You just have to do what you think is right and best for your facility and patients. If you let that be your guide, then in the end you will be successful.

From the moment I went to JFK Medical Center I knew it was an amazing place. To think that for that moment of time we were at the center of the world's attention and that we probably had a hand in saving countless lives is really humbling.

Interviewer: What upcoming likely events have you prepared for?

PDR: I was the CEO of St. Joseph Hospital in Houston in September of 2008, when our community was hit by Hurricane Ike. I had been so passionate about preparation for disasters and crises that we brought in our disaster consultant to help us set up the command center and instruct and evaluate our processes of managing through the preparation, the storm, and its aftermath. Although we found many things to improve, I think our team executed the plan flawlessly. We had little damage, no injuries, sheltered 700 staff members and their families, had a patient census of nearly 300, and never ceased normal operations during the entire event.

Interviewer: What did you do specifically to prepare your facility for likely events?

PDR: We had a disaster preparedness consultant who helped us refine and improve our plans. We conducted drills even on off hours and weekends, and made significant improvements to our communication systems, our command center, and our response readiness. In addition, our facility was set up to be a major triage facility in the event of a significant disaster. In fact, the ED has a self-contained air system where we can totally isolate or quarantine the department, and the entire five-floor parking garage can be converted into a triage facility in very short order.

Interviewer: What are the most important leadership characteristics that helped you to prepare for and respond to this event?

PDR: The culture that you as a leader create in your organization is one of the most important factors in successful management of a catastrophic event. If you are open, visible, and responsive and have developed public trust and confidence in your facility, you will excel in your response. During the hurricane, I personally sent out emails to the staff to reassure them and give them damage updates and progress reports. I encouraged the chaplains to hold prayer sessions, and at one point we held a large mass asking for strength and guidance during the storm. As trite as it sounds, you need to give your team what they need to get you through the event: information, reassurance, visibility, humor, calmness, and focus.

Interviewer: What were the personal consequences for you or your leadership staff from responding to this event?

PDR: I am not sure you ever really get over one of these events, especially if you or people you know are personally affected. In a hurricane or any other kind of disaster, many of your staff, your family, and your friends may well be victims themselves. Do not underestimate your own and your staff's spiritual and emotional needs during and after the event.

An Early Careerist's Perspective of Disaster Preparedness

Interview with Windsor Westbrook Sherrill, PhD, associate professor, Department of Health Sciences, Clemson University, Clemson, South Carolina

Interviewer: What has been your experience in dealing with disasters?

Windsor Westbrook Sherrill (WWS): As an administrative resident at a large academic medical center, I had the fortunate experience of being trained in disaster preparation during my residency program. I was able to work with the administrators responsible for disaster preparation as well as with the partner organizations preparing for disaster drills and exercises.

Disaster preparation is a critical competency that is often overlooked in administrative training for early careerists. Residents and new administrators are in a unique position to learn about disaster preparation, so organizations should take advantage of this opportunity as often as possible.

The community in which I trained had a comprehensive, coordinated approach to disaster planning. A large veterans' hospital was one of the community providers, and this facility served as the organizational arm for all healthcare organizations participating in disaster planning. As such, our organization's preparation for disasters was facilitated by a community-wide approach to disaster planning. The exercises were critical in developing administrative and clinical comfort with disaster situations. When an actual disaster occurred that involved a relatively large influx of patients, our facility was prepared, and the local providers were engaged in a partnership that facilitated the efficient processing of patients and response to the crisis.

Interviewer: Did the ownership/corporate structure of your hospital affect your response or participation in these planning and preparedness activities?

WWS: Interestingly, the various healthcare organizations who worked cooperatively on disaster preparation were otherwise staunch competitors. In the local community, a large academic medical center, a large community hospital, a military hospital, a medium-sized for-profit institution, and a small rehabilitation hospital worked together on the disaster exercise preparations. One of the most effective elements was having outside observers in each facility assess preparation and response. These observers typically came from competitor hospitals, but worked as allies on the task of improving disaster preparation for the community. This had the benefit of combining the talents of several organizations to improve community preparation, but also provided an opportunity for organizations that typically functioned as competitors to work cooperatively on a larger issue.

Interviewer: Describe the characteristics of your organization's "disaster culture" and how you might change the culture for future disaster response.

WWS: The individual organizations working on disaster preparation had to overcome the culture of competition that is typically a hallmark of healthcare. Internal to our facilities, disaster drills provided an opportunity for individuals at all levels of the organization to assume temporary leadership roles in jobs such as running a triage area or leading communication between components of the organization. It was rewarding to see the organization become flexible enough to transcend the usual organizational structure and form a matrix of teams and leaders to achieve effective disaster response.

Interviewer: How did you communicate internally and externally during this disaster?

WWS: All individuals in the disaster exercises participated with ham radio operators who were important to the drill process throughout the community. Exercise leaders at each treatment and triage area had hand-held radios which were stored in our disaster areas and always charged.

Interviewer: What was the biggest challenge to your employees and your medical staff during these exercises?

WWS: Because exercises occurred at least yearly, the staff became accustomed to the process, and was able to continue regular operations while participating in drills or exercises. One of the most rewarding aspects of the drill process was the emotional "charge" that every individual involved in the process felt. Environmental services workers became temporary transporters; physicians from one area of the institution would become triage leaders; individuals would assume roles different from their day-to-day activities but that also took advantage of their unique skills. As such, the exercise process was rewarding to individuals and beneficial to the organization.

Interviewer: What agencies, individuals, or organizations were most helpful? Did any impede your ability to respond?

WWS: Our institution worked directly with three major medical centers in the community as well as with the Army medical center to set up a regional disaster exercise each year, an arrangement which was particularly effective.

Interviewer: What did you do that you feel was right?

WWS: The use of live "patients" for the exercise procedures was critical to establishing a true test of the disaster response of an organization. This was achieved by another community partnership. The disaster scenario and patient profiles were prepared by the community-wide disaster response team. Individuals serving as patients were soldiers from the local military base, an arrangement facilitated by the military hospital. A local theater company and makeup artists were recruited to assist with transforming soldiers into the injured disaster victims, and "victims" were coached in role playing their symptoms and diagnoses.

Interviewer: What did you learn about yourself, your team, and your facility?

WWS: I have never seen our facility so energized and unified. It was professionally rewarding to see individuals from all departments working together to transport, triage, and treat patients.

Interviewer: What things would you do differently? How has the hospital changed after this event?

WWS: Leadership is critical to the value placed on disaster planning and the exercise processes by the organization. A community-wide approach required input and commitment from all players, and this can only be achieved by leaders who place value on the process of preparation and testing. The follow-up evaluation assessment and after-action review of the exercises were always beneficial to each participating organization, and they typically resulted in changes to internal policies and increased preparation within each organization.

Involving administrative and medical residents in disaster preparedness adds a great deal to the educational experience and preparation in health services.

Interviewer: Were there unexpected consequences of this experience?

WWS: As an early careerist, participating in a leadership role in the planning and implementation processes for major disaster preparedness helped me develop leadership skills and confidence in disaster preparation. I have repeatedly called on these experiences in other organizations and settings.

Interviewer: What surprised or shocked you about your experience?

WWS: I distinctly recall being surprised by my personal sense of accomplishment and the pride of our organization after a successful disaster drill or exercise. There was quite literally an emotional response within our organization, and this has had an effect on me throughout my career in health services. I saw that employees value the experience and feeling of preparation for disaster situations that can arise, and individuals appreciate and take pride in opportunities to develop preparedness.

Interviewer: What advice would you give for those who will face similar situations in the future?

WWS: Involve early careerist administrators and clinicians in disaster preparedness training. This specific skill set is one that either can be acquired through disaster drills, exercises, and preparedness training, or through a "hit or miss" experience in actual disaster situations. Individuals trained early in their careers will be comfortable with situations that might occur throughout their careers. Disaster preparation is a critical competency that is often missing in administrative training for early careerists. New administrators and managers-in-training are in a unique position to learn about disaster preparation, so organizations should work to incorporate related training and exposure to disaster preparation as much as possible.

Interviewer: What are the most important leadership characteristics that helped you to assume a leadership role in preparing and responding to potential disaster events?

WWS: Disaster preparation, drills, and exercises help individuals develop confidence in situations of uncertainty. No two disaster scenarios should be set up the same way, just as no two disaster situations will ever have the same circumstances. The key to disaster planning and training is to develop the skills that are needed to make good decisions during a disaster situation. Only training and disaster modeling can prepare individuals and organizations for occurrences that strain the healthcare system.

Devastation on Galveston Island: The University of Texas Medical Branch at Galveston and Hurricane Ike

Interview with David L. Callender, MD, FACS, president, the University of Texas Medical Branch at Galveston; and Michael J. Megna, FACHE, associate vice president and institutional emergency preparedness officer, the University of Texas Medical Branch at Galveston

In September 2008, Hurricane Ike wreaked havoc in the Gulf of Mexico, hitting Galveston Island especially hard. The University of Texas Medical Branch (UTMB) hospital, one of the premier academic medical centers in the country and a vital part of the Galveston community, sustained great damage. UTMB President Dr. David Callender and Institutional Emergency Preparedness Officer Michael Megna describe the experience of saving a state legend.

Interviewer: What has been your experience in dealing with disasters?

David L. Callender (DLC): Before becoming president of the University of Texas Medical Branch at Galveston in 2007, I served as chief executive officer of the UCLA hospital system and, prior to that, as executive vice president and chief operating officer at the University of Texas MD Anderson Cancer Center. In each of these positions, I played a key role in planning for a wide range of emergency situations and in executing responses to actual events.

Although UCLA experienced no serious catastrophe during my term there, we were in a constant state of readiness to respond to environmental disasters such as earthquakes and fires, major utilities failures, and man-made emergencies such as bomb threats. Tropical Storm Allison struck Southeast Texas during my term at MD Anderson Cancer Center, causing major flooding and significant damage in the Houston area. Among the many health institutions in the Texas Medical

Center (including Baylor College of Medicine, Texas Children's Hospital, Memorial Hermann, and the University of Texas Health Sciences Center at Houston), MD Anderson was the only one that suffered virtually no damage—the fortuitous result of new flood management gear that was fully operational within minutes of the decision to engage it. I have been at UTMB for approximately two years and, with tightly knit leadership and incident command teams, helped steer the institution through the 2008 hurricane season (which included the devastating Hurricane Ike). I have helped ensure that UTMB is prepared for emergencies ranging from fires, utilities failures, and laboratory incidents on campus to petrochemical explosions, epidemics, and other mass catastrophes.

Michael J. Megna (MJM): In addition to my duties on the hospital administration team, I have been working in an emergency preparedness capacity during the last ten years. I am responsible for developing and revising our emergency operations plan as well as the disaster preparedness portion of The Joint Commission requirements. Over the last four years, I have been working to improve our evacuation and command center plans, a process that has been accelerated because of hands-on experience during hurricanes Rita and Ike.

Interviewer: Please describe what happened during Hurricane Ike.

DLC: Hurricane Ike was the third most destructive hurricane to make landfall in the United States. It was the ninth named storm, fifth hurricane, and third major hurricane of the 2008 Atlantic hurricane season. Ike began as a tropical disturbance off the coast of Africa near the end of August, became a Category 4 hurricane with maximum sustained winds of 145 mph the morning of September 4, and made landfall east of Galveston, Texas, as a Category 2 hurricane (with a storm surge more characteristic of a Category 4 storm) on September 13 at 2:10 am.

In anticipation of the storm, UTMB began a phased shutdown of research activities (including those taking place in maximum-containment laboratories built for the safe study of some of the most serious infectious threats to human health), canceled classes and released students, canceled clinic visits and elective surgeries, discharged hospital patients able to return home safely, evacuated over 300 patients to facilities located beyond the storm's path, released nonessential employees, relocated academic and vital support functions (e.g., finance and information technology) to distant secure locations, and secured campus facilities according to our established emergency plans.

Ike's storm surge flooded more than 1 million square feet of first-floor space on the UTMB campus, with flood levels ranging from a few inches in the university library to approximately eight feet in historic "Old Red," the state's first medical school building. John Sealy Hospital, the hub of UTMB's clinical care complex, also sustained serious flooding. The pharmacy, blood bank, food services, and sterile processing areas—essential elements of inpatient and trauma care—were lost as a result. The loss of these critical ancillary services also caused the shutdown of UTMB's elite Level 1 Trauma Center—one of only three in the region; the trauma center is scheduled to reopen as a Level 3 facility in the summer of 2009, almost one year after the storm. Research laboratories and classroom space, including the gross anatomy lab, also suffered significant damage. Imaging equipment, linear accelerators, patient simulation equipment, and other critical resources were also lost.

Interviewer: Prior to this event, how had your facility prepared for responding to a major disaster or catastrophic event? How well do you feel your facility responded to this event?

DLC: Campus-wide preparation and training for hurricanes and other emergencies take place on a routine basis, consistent with UTMB's institutional disaster preparedness policy. In fact, a hurricane simulation disaster drill was conducted about two weeks before Hurricane Ike. Vital and extensive communications channels are established and rigorously maintained with the state's Emergency Operations Center and local/regional emergency response teams during times of regional or state emergencies. A comprehensive incident command structure, with institutional and departmental emergency response plans, is firmly in place—along with an annual process for designating essential personnel needed to help the institution prepare for, respond to, and recover from a disaster. Disaster insurance coverage is secured by the University of Texas System for its campuses in the Houston–Galveston region, and contracts for disaster response services are set through UT System's Office of Risk Management.

In terms of Hurricane Ike, stocks of fuel, water, food, and medical supplies, as well as alternative power sources, were available on campus or staged at nearby locations in advance of the storm. Core business recovery functions were relocated off campus consistent with existing business continuity plans. Laboratories were shut down "by the book." Hurricanes Rita and Katrina changed everyone's thinking about the need to evacuate patients and employees to safety, and our skilled staff conducted the second complete patient evacuation in our 118-year history without a hitch.

It's doubtful the institution could have been any more prepared with regard to the readiness of personnel and supplies. I rate UTMB's preparedness for the event as a 7 or 8 out of 10 because our facilities and those in this region of the Texas coast were not adequately protected from the major storm surge that was significantly greater and more destructive than those associated with previous hurricanes or a typical Category 2 or 3 storm. In fact, the use of the Saffir-Simpson hurricane classification scale has changed as a result of Hurricane Ike. Our campus lacked an adequate comprehensive flood management system to mitigate the risk of such a storm surge. Previously, such a flood management system was felt to be prohibitively expensive from a cost/benefit perspective. Obviously, we and many others learned much from Hurricane Ike.

Interviewer: Did the ownership/corporate structure of your hospital affect your response to this event?

DLC: The mutual support agreements in place through the University of Texas System helped us establish and sustain a comprehensive and effective response and were extraordinarily helpful. Also, single institutional governance of the education, research, clinical, and business enterprises enabled us to evaluate emerging challenges and opportunities and to make decisions quickly. Unfortunately, being a state institution that is not affiliated with a major private health system meant we lacked "deep pockets" to fall back on right after the storm. As a result, although we were able to reopen many of our outpatient clinics on the mainland within a few days or weeks of the storm, there was no alternative hospital space for our physicians and nurses to provide inpatient care, and no way to quickly replace lost clinical revenue. To preserve critical cash reserves to support the costs of recovery, we reduced our workforce from approximately 12,500 full-time equivalents (FTE) to about 10,000 FTE two months after the storm. This was an incredibly painful step during a very difficult time, but was felt to be necessary to allow us to have a chance to recover.

MJM: Being part of the University of Texas System was a blessing during the recovery process as it allowed us the mutual aid agreements and additional resources that might not have been available to us if we were a private entity. The affiliation also allowed us to speak directly to state-level emergency operations officials rather than local entities. These agreements also ensured that UTMB was not competing for resources that were also being requested by local governments or private businesses in Galveston County.

Interviewer: Do you feel you had the right culture to sustain you through this disaster? If so, describe the characteristics of your culture. If not, why and how would you or how have you changed the culture for future response?

DLC: UTMB's doors had been open for less than a decade when the Great Storm of 1900 (with an estimated death toll of 6,000 people) devastated

Galveston Island. When the University of Texas System Board of Regents received a telegram the day following the storm describing six feet of water in the basement of Old Red and asking if the medical school should open, they responded that UT "stops for no storm." That same resilience, sense of family, and everyday heroism—or willingness to put the needs of others before one's own—has continued since 1900 and has sustained UTMB through every adversity it has faced, including Hurricane Ike. In short, UTMB's people remain committed to living up to the legacy of stopping for no storm.

MJM: During Hurricane Rita, we learned that the visibility of the leadership team and transparent and decisive decision making were key to a successful disaster recovery effort. During and following Hurricane Ike, Dr. Callender and the other members of our incident command staff were available and very visible in the recovery effort, which was a reassurance to our employees.

Interviewer: How did you communicate internally/externally during this disaster?

DLC: The audiences with which we needed to communicate included faculty, staff, students (and parents), patients, alumni, donors, elected officials, the University of Texas System, peer/partner institutions, state and federal agencies, and the public at large through the news media. Throughout preparation, response, and recovery we communicated via the Web (internal and external sites), email, FirstCall (a multimedia emergency notification system including voice, email, and text options representing a "push" approach implemented in the wake of the Virginia Tech tragedy), alert phone lines (local and 800 numbers), and the news media (i.e., advisories, public service announcements, interviews, and press conferences). Essential personnel staffed the emergency operations center in shifts, and meetings took place according to schedule several times a day, followed by updates via all available communication channels. In the critical days just before, during, and immediately after the storm, faculty and staff met in the cafeteria of the John Sealy Hospital and then the Texas Department of Criminal Justice Hospital (after flooding destroyed the John Sealy cafeteria), where the incident commander (a function shared by the president, the head of the health system, and the institutional emergency preparedness officer) provided status reports and reviewed plans using a bullhorn. We were without reliable phone, cell, and email service for approximately 24 hours after Ike made landfall. We used a persistent Web server and an automated "mirror" email system (an off-site location where the Web server and all email are duplicated for backup) established at another UT System institution, but could not access those immediately after the storm because of network issues. Until the persistent Web server was functional, we were able to communicate with our external communities via a contracted blog-based website identified after Hurricane Rita. Additionally, our partners in the State Emergency Operations Center were also an invaluable link to the outside world. We attempted to use any communication channel that might be available to us in the first few days after the storm. At one point, a member of our media relations staff actually got on his bike and went on a hunt for reporters, who followed him back to UTMB and were able to get out the news that the university had sustained significant damage but had weathered the storm. We also made good use of low-tech easel pads for posting notices and passing personal memos from worried family members along to on-site staff. This year, we are evaluating the effectiveness of social media (namely, Twitter and Facebook) in emergency communications, particularly those aimed at faculty, staff, and students.

MJM: Face-to-face meetings along with the Internet were the cornerstones of our communication. Our internal communication systems all failed during the recovery. Telephones, cell phones, two-way radios, our emergency backup, and law enforcement emergency radio were all out of commission at one point or another. To keep our staff informed, we held briefings during meal times. These briefings provided a good opportunity to update the staff and allow them to ask questions. Externally, we were extremely lucky to have public information officers who were able to use the media effectively. Our information services group deployed staff to Arlington, Texas, to operate a persistent failover computer network (a redundant or standby network to which the system automatically switches), which at one point was used to support communications in Galveston.

Interviewer: What was the biggest challenge to your employees and your medical staff during this disaster?

DLC: The environment itself (e.g., the lack of running water with loss of flushing toilets and sewage service; the loss of air conditioning, elevators, and lights; and the loss of food preparation facilities) was probably the most significant challenge to safety and our ability to protect and preserve our facilities and programs. Additionally, the overwhelming amount of things that had to be done right away to preserve and protect UTMB and to begin putting the institution back on its feet was daunting. Also, a large number of faculty and staff suffered personal losses and were faced with the ongoing challenge of finding alternative housing, filing FEMA claims, and coping with psychological stress. Uncertainty about the future took a heavy toll over the course of time, as did the previously mentioned reduction in force, which resulted in additional responsibilities for people already working at full capacity and grieving for colleagues who had lost their jobs.

Interviewer: What agencies, individuals, or organizations were most helpful? Did any impede your ability to respond?

DLC: UTMB's planning, response, and recovery efforts benefited immensely from the support of a host of agencies, organizations, and individuals almost too numerous to count. These include:

- Federal and state legislators and elected officials
- Federal government agencies (e.g., FEMA, Centers for Disease Control, National Institutes of Health, FBI)
- Federal response teams (i.e., Disaster Medical Assistance Teams and others such as Disaster Mortuary Assistance Teams [DMORTs] and Veterinary Medical Assistance Teams [VMATs])
- State of Texas agencies (e.g., Governor's Office/Division of Emergency Management State Operations Center, Texas Legislature, Department of State Health Services, Health and Human Services Commission, Catastrophic Medical Operations Center, National Guard)
- City and county emergency operations centers, government officials, and community leaders
- University of Texas System regents, administrators, and numerous UT academic and health sciences institutions
- Other Texas universities (e.g., Texas A&M University at Galveston and Baylor College of Medicine) and universities throughout the nation
- Numerous regional and state healthcare partners/providers
- Alumni, students, and Galveston residents who advocated effectively for funding during the 81st Texas Legislative Session to support UTMB's recovery
- Multiple philanthropic organizations and individuals who contributed more than $1 million to help with UTMB student recovery
- Numerous professional organizations

MJM: In addition to the entities Dr. Callender has mentioned, our various contractors were phenomenal. At one point, we had more than 1,500 people cleaning a damaged area of more than 1.2 million square feet. I found that no entities really impeded us to the point that it hindered our recovery efforts. In fact, the University of Texas, and state and federal officials who visited our campus were quite impressed by the non-UTMB personnel working side by side with our staff to get the job done.

Interviewer: What do you wish you had known before this event?

DLC: I wish we would have known the extent of the storm surge and probable damage with ensuing effect on our operations. Based on UTMB's experience with previous storms, we mistakenly thought that we should be prepared to resume most hospital operations immediately after the storm. Although our emergency staff provided care to approximately 120 individuals who arrived during or immediately after the storm, we would not have kept approximately 250 caregivers on-site had we known that the storm surge would be so great or the campus so stricken. In the future, if we anticipate a storm of this magnitude, we intend to lock down the campus and ride out the storm with the minimum number of people needed to safeguard the facilities. We also intend to take physical fitness into account when designating essential personnel in the future, given the primitive conditions and physical challenges we faced in the wake of Ike.

MJM: I wish we would have better understood that the areas we thought were safe were actually very susceptible to flooding. We thought the mechanical systems would function throughout the storm, but found that our transfer switches were more vulnerable than initially thought. Underground utilities such as steam, water, and telephone lines were much more damaged than anticipated. We also discovered unexpected secondary consequences from Hurricane Ike. For example, we did not foresee the damage that would be incurred when the elevator lines were submerged in salt water. Half of our 134 elevators were out of service.

Interviewer: What did you do that you feel was right?

DLC: Capable institutional leaders functioning in concert led to the quickness of our response and the speed of our recovery. Our communications strategies—built on regular, timely, informative, and honest updates, in person and via other available outlets—worked well in what can best be described as fluid and dynamic circumstances. People appreciated hearing our assessment of a given situation and what we were doing to address it. Those updates also served to underscore that measurable progress was being made. Finally, we coined the phrase "protect and preserve" in the days immediately following the storm—the phrase became a mantra or rallying cry that kept people focused on the task at hand and helped them understand the importance of their individual contributions to the recovery process.

MJM: Making definitive decisions and sticking to a timeline are two of the more important characteristics of how we responded to Hurricane Ike. Our proactive nature led us to begin working with the state five days before Hurricane Ike made landfall. Making the decision to evacuate our patients was extremely difficult, but ultimately we realized it was the safest course of action. Inviting consultation and expert opinion from different organizations and individuals proved to be very helpful as well.

Interviewer: What three things would you do differently? How has the hospital changed after this event?

DLC: As noted previously, we are crafting a new plan that describes who stays on-site during a disaster. We also will build a better plan for communicating the new practice locations for our healthcare providers in the event UTMB's existing clinical sites and operations are disrupted by a catastrophe. Additionally, we plan to adjust our communications strategies based on our Ike experiences so that we have access to the greatest number of two-way communications channels to keep us linked to the outside world. Finally, we are raising critical functions and infrastructure and building flood management systems that will allow us to avoid such substantial facilities and functional losses with future storms.

MJM: To reinforce Dr. Callender's comments, we are working on a plan that would allow us to have fewer people on campus during a disaster. During Hurricane Ike, 550 employees stayed to help keep the hospital operational. We are hoping to reduce that number and put more people on the northern side of Houston with a plan to get them back once it is proven safe to do so. We also recognize that people involved in the recovery effort need more relief than initially projected. They should be able to physically leave the work site and go to an environment where they are able to relax. Reopening the hospital is another aspect of recovery that we would handle differently. Rather than rushing the reentry process, we would make sure all aspects of the operation are accounted for and would support the resumption of services without a secondary failure. You cannot recover too slowly.

Interviewer: Were there unexpected consequences of this experience? If so, what were they?

DLC: We didn't predict the massive amount of money (more than $1 billion) needed to support UTMB's recovery or the fact that no single source had the financial capacity to address the need. Fortunately, another unanticipated consequence of the storm was the reawakened and expanded appreciation of the vital contributions UTMB makes to the health and well-being of its home community, the region at large, and the state as a whole.

Interviewer: What surprised or shocked you about your experience?

DLC: As noted before, the vulnerability of our facilities and the magnitude of the costs involved in recovery came as something of a shock. That said, UTMB's recovery has gone faster and farther than that of many other institutions faced with a disaster of this magnitude, and everyone involved has much for which to be proud as they consider the response to the events of September 2008.

MJM: The emergency planning world drills you on planning and responding to "what if" situations. The multiple failures we experienced were unexpected but should have been anticipated.

Interviewer: What advice would you give for those who will face similar situations in the future?

DLC: First, have a comprehensive, all-hazards plan, then prepare and drill for emergency situations. Because emergency situations rarely unfold according to plan—during Ike we found ourselves frequently saying that we'd moved beyond plan A, to plan B, to plan C, and so forth, and were now at letter H—practice is essential to the creation of the nimble and imaginative responses required in the face of a disaster. Those in command must also provide an environment that allows people to use their best judgment and take appropriate actions within the overall response plan parameters.

MJM: Have a good emergency operations plan in place. Make sure your people know and understand this plan. When practicing and conducting drills, take your scenario to a dimension you've not planned for before. You may know your vulnerabilities, but what about your city's vulnerabilities or other stakeholder vulnerabilities? In the course of your exercises, know who your key people are and what their capabilities are. Make sure they are in the right job.

Interviewer: What did you learn about yourself, your team, and your facility?

DLC: My primary focus was on the functioning of the incident command and institutional leadership teams; the well-being of our faculty, staff, and students; the preservation of our programs; and the integrity of our physical plant. While I didn't spend a great deal of time reflecting on my own responses, the storm underscored for me the resolute determination of our UTMB family members and their inspiring ability to come together and work for the good of all. I also learned just how vulnerable our facilities are to major flooding. Given the imperative to recover operations as quickly as possible following a disaster, we are determined to markedly reduce that risk in the coming years.

MJM: People were tasked with assignments and worked with minimal supervision. They knew to ask for help if needed. Our employees and those involved in the recovery effort showed incredible strength, ingenuity, and resourcefulness. We all learned quickly how to succeed in jobs we had never done before and accomplished some incredible things on the first try.

MJM: We are devoting a great deal of training time to and conducting exercises around emerging infections—primarily influenza—and the likely scenario of large numbers of people in need of medical care while having a much reduced workforce as a result of the same infection.

Interviewer: What are the most important leadership characteristics that helped you to prepare for and respond to this event?

DLC: I've been fortunate to have great teachers and mentors in the course of my professional and personal life. They taught me that leaders help those around them manage the attendant stress and tension of a crisis while generating creative responses to challenges. It's important to maintain humor and hope. It's also important to respect the need of those affected to be tired, angry, overwhelmed, frustrated, and sad—in short, to be human. Leaders must recognize limitations in times of crisis, understanding that while most people are capable of heroic acts, they are not superhuman. Leaders should also trust their own instincts and those of the people with whom they work. Finally, in times of emergency, leaders ask questions and provide direction to get people to expand their thinking beyond the losses of the moment to the first or next steps of the recovery process.

Interviewer: What were the personal consequences for you or your leadership staff from responding to this event?

DLC: The large-scale reduction in force that was necessary to preserve UTMB's limited cash reserves for investment in recovery operations was the single most disturbing and demoralizing consequence of the storm for leaders, faculty, staff, and students alike. UTMB is a cornerstone of the Galveston community and by far the largest employer in the county. As a result, the threat of closing the institution, and the impact of the reduction in force and reduced clinical services, was devastating. Luckily, thanks to widespread support for the institution from our federal and state legislators, alumni, and many friends, we survived and are now beginning the rebuilding and renovation of our facilities and programs. There is great confidence that the process will result in an even stronger, more successful institution.

MJM: There were individuals involved in running major aspects of the organization whose homes were destroyed. Several storm-related deaths occurred within the UTMB family, which incredibly affected our staff. The storm also exacerbated stress and other medical conditions. I have great admiration for those who stuck with their jobs to bring the organization back online even while they were dealing with these and other issues.

Flooding in the Lone Star State: Texas Children's Hospital and Tropical Storm Allison

Interview with Randall Wright, FACHE, chief operating officer, Texas Children's Hospital, Houston

In the early summer months of 2001, Tropical Storm (TS) Allison struck the Texas coastline with ferocity. Houston received the majority of Allison's fury, recording 37 inches of rain in only two days. The Texas Medical Center, the largest medical complex in the world, experienced massive flooding that threatened the hospitals that call that area home. Texas Children's Hospital (TCH) is one of those hospitals. With over 700 licensed pediatric beds, the hospital required a coordinated response and effort on behalf of its leaders and employees to survive. Randall Wright, chief operating officer at TCH, leads us through the event, describing his response and preparedness before, during, and after Allison.

Interviewer: Please describe what happened during TS Allison.

Randall Wright (RW): TS Allison occurred in early June of 2001 and dumped heavy rains on areas surrounding the Texas Medical Center. While the largest storm occurred on a Friday evening and continued through Saturday morning, there were heavy rains throughout the entire week. On the Tuesday prior to the flood, our organization called in our command center team because of the heavy rain, but no significant flooding occurred that night. On Friday evening, the administrator on call, in conjunction with the chief nursing officer, determined there was potential for rain to disrupt our normal business operations and that it was important to have the management team on-site. They called all of the command center team to report to the campus and be available to help manage the event. Most of our teams were on-site by approximately 8:00 pm that evening, and we opened our command center.

Our first priority was to manage staffing in the clinical areas and assign personnel to monitor areas that could be affected by the storm. TCH changes shifts for clinical areas at 7:00 am and 7:00 pm, and because of the way the storm progressed, the majority of our staff were on-site for the normal shift change when the storm hit. We were able to monitor the intensity of the storm through the Internet and through communication with emergency preparedness agencies. Between midnight and 1:00 am, the Braes Bayou and drainage system around the Texas Medical Center reached capacity and the water level began to rise in the streets. At that time, we closed all flood doors and placed flood logs to protect garage entrances. At approximately 2:00 am, normal power was lost, and emergency generators started automatically. We did have some difficulty with one emergency transfer switch that provided support for elevators, a problem that took the facilities team about two hours to resolve. During that time, vertical movement of people and supplies occurred through the stairwells. At approximately 4:00 am, we received word that The Methodist Hospital had significant flooding, and that water was flowing from The Methodist Hospital through the tunnel into St. Luke's Hospital and Texas Children's Hospital. It became clear that areas outside our flood doors would be lost to flood water. St. Luke's staff realized that they would lose both power and communications and began moving patients down from the upper floors. As the water migrated through the tunnels, the lowest point it could reach was a three-level garage underground, and water was purposefully channeled to that location as a holding area.

The following morning, a support team built a temporary retaining wall to contain any flood water that might flow between interconnected parking garages. As water receded, we were able to initiate pumping operations to pull the water out of the basement areas. We also began working with our adjacent hospitals, in particular, The Methodist Hospital, where they had lost significant ability to care for patients because of damage to power, air conditioning, and other systems. One of our recently vacated patient care units was turned into an adult nursing area for The Methodist Hospital. They also shared some of our operating rooms to provide surgical venues for their patients. All told, TCH suffered approximately $3 million in damage as a result of TS Allison, but no significant interruption of patient services occurred.

Interviewer: Prior to this event, how had your facility prepared for responding to a major disaster or catastrophic event? How well do you feel your facility responded to this event?

RW: We conduct regular drills and exercises on various scenarios, and flooding in the Texas Medical Center and hurricanes in Texas are part of that training. We were fortunate that we called the alert approximately three days before the tropical storm hit. This provided us an opportunity to review all issues associated with staffing and availability of supplies, among other matters. I believe our response to Allison was excellent. All major areas that could have been protected were, and overall patient care activities functioned as expected.

Interviewer: Did the ownership/corporate structure of your hospital affect your response to this event?

RW: I am not sure that our response would have been dramatically different if we had been under another sort of ownership or structure, but certainly the link to community resources was critical. In my opinion, the board involvement has greatly benefited TCH in planning activities. We have multiple board members who are business leaders in our community. They take an active role in protecting the integrity of our structure, and in this example, they led the decision-making process to invest in upgraded flood doors that would ensure the safety of our facilities. Also, following the event, many board members were on-site and, because of their standing in the community, were able to provide access to things that we would not have had normally—particularly standby generators and pumps.

Interviewer: Do you feel that you had the right culture to sustain you through this disaster? If so, describe the characteristics of your culture. If not, why and how would you or how have you changed the culture for future disaster response?

RW: I believe children's hospitals have a different culture compared to many adult facilities, and TCH is unique even among children's hospitals. It is a committed and caring group of individuals who chose to work with children for very specific reasons. In addition, our administrative team, led by CEO Mark Wallace, has strong management skills and excellent rapport and communication. Even in the midst of the crisis, we employed professional, courteous, and thoughtful communication amongst individuals and in our coordination of staff efforts. Once the flood receded, we had a unique opportunity to work with our neighbors to reach out and provide support in their time of need.

Interviewer: How did you communicate internally and externally during this disaster?

RW: TS Allison was a very short-term event for TCH, basically starting Friday evening and winding down by Sunday evening. During the storm, access to the Internet for weather information and phone communication with our neighboring institutions was important. Following the Allison event, the Texas Medical

Center took the lead in working with all the organizations to ensure there were common guidelines and parameters used for decisions regarding installation of flood protection and when emergency measures should be activated. During long-term events such as Hurricane Ike (2008) and the H1N1 outbreak (2009), internal communication was a priority. Our public affairs staff is integrated into our planning teams and manages all communication.

Interviewer: What was the biggest challenge to your employees and your medical staff during this disaster?

RW: During Allison, the biggest issue for staff was probably the disruption of normal life. Our process is to assign staff to different teams for disaster events, and we continue to refine that model, which allows individuals to know what their responsibilities will be. This provides them with a format to manage their personal matters and prioritize their time.

Interviewer: What agencies, individuals, or organizations were most helpful? Did any impede your ability to respond?

RW: We were fortunate that one of our employees is an active participant in the regional disaster management program. She actually sits in their command center during emergencies and provides links to TCH. The biggest challenge that we continue to find is the relationship with the patient community and, particularly, those special-needs patients who require support but not necessarily hospitalization, such as ventilator-dependent and dialysis patients. Having a regional solution will be important. Obviously, the public works agencies, Reliant Energy (electricity) and City of Houston (water and sewage), are extremely important for hospitals. During Hurricane Ike in 2008, we benefited from all the effort that had gone into preparing for the hurricane—underground power, multiple trunk lines, and so forth—which worked well. We had no power outages during the storm. We were also fortunate that we never lost water pressure or sewage during the storm, but still anticipate that these will be points of vulnerability in the future.

Interviewer: What do you wish you had known before this event?

RW: The biggest issue was the response of our neighboring facilities during disasters. It is very easy to get so locked into your own response and your own plan that you lose track of what is going on around you that may ultimately affect you. The development of links to companion organizations and the community is important.

Interviewer: What did you do right?

RW: The decision to activate the emergency team early is important. It may mean more false events, but at the same time, it reduces the potential for a true event where you are not properly prepared.

Interviewer: What three things would you do differently? How has the hospital changed after this event?

RW: Communication with our peer institutions has been dramatically improved. Second, we have moved more aggressively to install flood doors and flood protection in all of our areas and increased flood protection in our new facilities. Finally, as we have become more experienced with the Incident Command System, we have identified new ways to strengthen and manage various areas of emergency response. For example, with the development of the H1N1 flu outbreak in the spring of 2009, the Planning and Operations Groups of the Incident Command System took the lead and we did not bring up the entire incident command process.

Interviewer: Were there unexpected consequences of this experience? If so, what were they?

RW: Providing support for our neighbors following the event was not anticipated. Being able to share operating rooms and inpatient services with them proved very satisfying.

Interviewer: What surprised or shocked you about your experience?

RW: In hindsight, there were two things in particular. First was the realization that while we were managing the process at our particular campus, we lost track of what was happening in the community. It wasn't until approximately 24 to 36 hours later that we realized the extent of the flooding and the amount of loss and suffering that hit different areas of our community and, in some cases, our employees. Second, I was shocked at the amount of damage at some of our neighbor institutions. Hundreds of millions of dollars in damage was caused by the flood. One large hospital was closed for several weeks, and others had their capabilities reduced during the several months required for repairs.

Interviewer: What advice would you give for those who will face similar situations in the future?

RW: First, take a step back and think critically about the potential exposures to your organization. In this instance, the continuing threat of flooding in the Texas Medical Center was identified and an aggressive flood protection program prevented TCH from having significant losses. Second, realize that events that are unplanned and unexpected create needs that are unplanned and unexpected. I look back at the experiences with both Hurricane Katrina and Hurricane Rita. Katrina, in particular, brought thousands of individuals from New Orleans to Houston, and TCH became a major pediatric care provider for the evacuees. Rita, which followed four weeks later, created huge traffic and logistics issues that affected our community. In both instances, the events were not a scenario that we had anticipated, but our process for management of resources and decision making worked very well. We developed responses that met the immediate needs while maintaining the integrity of the patient care program at TCH. The message there would be, "Make sure your processes work so that the individuals who drive the Incident Command System can apply their skill set to whatever issue is at hand."

Interviewer: What did you learn about yourself, your team, and your facility?

RW: I learned that a strong leadership team is resourceful, resilient, and responsive. We were pleased that the proactive facilities measures worked as designed. We continue to improve the emergency response model to create redundancy. The leadership team has continued to refine the Incident Command System, and we now have teams assigned to each of the major areas, rooms assigned to support each of these groups, and have increased the depth of trained leaders on our teams.

Interviewer: What upcoming likely events have you prepared for?

RW: The experience in 2009 with H1N1 was a different scenario than the traditional bad weather phenomena. The effect on our laboratories, our staffing, our emergency room, and patient screening were all new experiences. We now have refined the processes that allow us to address that type of demand and have a new ER triage model to preserve the integrity of our inpatient base at the same time as we screen and treat those outpatients that may have infectious diseases.

Interviewer: What have you done specifically to prepare your facility for likely events?

RW: The key factor has been having a trained and experienced team and an Incident Command System that can respond to almost any event. Because of our experience with the H1N1 virus, we continue to find ways to improve the structure.

We also conduct exercises around events and have extended exercises to include the recovery process. Just before Hurricane Ike hit, we had been through a recovery exercise that proved very beneficial. It is always a challenge to model the impact of civil order during disasters, because we depend on local police departments for armed security. Based on the experience in New Orleans following Hurricane Katrina, we have identified resources that may be available in a disaster, but having access to the resources we need is still a concern. The team that Mark Wallace has in place is composed of strong leaders with excellent independent judgment. Having the authority and confidence to make timely decisions is critical. Simultaneously, the Incident Command System provides the overall guidance and coordination. Disaster preparedness and exercises feel like a burden, but we believe there is benefit to working through these examples and building a level of confidence in the response process.

Interviewer: What are the most important leadership characteristics that helped you to prepare for and respond to this event?

RW: Experience is important to responding quickly. In this context, having the vision to push the development of emergency planning and drills has created the experience level of the management team in responding to unplanned events. Traditional leadership traits such as dedication, humility, and creativity all have a place creating the culture that supports the management team during a time of crisis.

Interviewer: What were the personal consequences for you or your leadership staff from responding to this event?

RW: In all cases, we benefited from our experiences. In the nine years since I have been at TCH, we have been through one significant flood, the September 11, 2001, tragedy, multiple storm and hurricane preparations, three significant hurricane events, a significant flu outbreak, and numerous smaller events. These represent opportunities for the teams to show their resilience and creativity to respond to unusual events that could severely impact the mission of our organization. Because these events play out in real time, certainly much faster than the traditional business-planning model, they are valuable learning experiences. The TCH team has the belief and expectation that while events of this nature are never pleasant, with training and experience they have the ability to respond successfully.

Interviewer: Is there anything else you would like to include?

RW: The scale of a disaster is important to include in the preparedness process. In major events, at some point, the emphasis will shift from managing the event to managing the future of the organization in the environment to follow. We saw this phenomenon with both Hurricane Katrina, which left large numbers of evacuees in the Houston area, and with Hurricane Ike, which closed major hospitals in Galveston and also displaced people. The effect on patient volume, payer mix, and physician referrals will all drive the business for periods long beyond the disaster itself. The concept of business continuity is very real and should be part of the planning process.

Disasters in Arkansas: The Hospital's and Hospital Association's Viewpoint

Interview with Angela L. Richmond, FACHE, president/CEO, Community Medical Center of Izard County; Kirk Reamey, FACHE, CEO, Ozark Health; and Beth Ingram, vice president, Arkansas Hospital Association

In recent years, Arkansas has been no stranger to catastrophic disasters. In 2008, an F4 tornado tore through the north central region, leaving a 123-mile-long disaster zone in its wake. In January 2009, an ice storm hit the same region, downing power lines, disabling utilities, and decimating tree limbs. Two Arkansas hospital CEOs, Kirk Reamey and Angela Richmond, describe their experiences in dealing with these disasters. Beth Ingram of the Arkansas Hospital Association also gives her insight.

Interviewer: What has been your experience in dealing with disasters?

Angela L. Richmond (ALR): Our area was fortunate to be narrowly missed by a devastating tornado and massive flood in 2008. However, that luck ended when freezing rain ran across north central Arkansas beginning on Monday evening, January 26, 2009. By Tuesday afternoon up to three inches of ice had fallen, decimating tree limbs, downing electric lines, and snapping utility poles for miles. Outside, you felt like you were in an ice palace. At the time of the ice storm, I was the CEO of two critical access hospitals: the Community Medical Center of Izard County (CMC) in Calico Rock, Arkansas, and Fulton County Hospital (FCH) in Salem, Arkansas. Both facilities lost their electric power and telephone lines early Tuesday morning, cell phone lines were lost by Tuesday evening, and Calico Rock lost its water supply on Tuesday evening.

Kirk Reamey (KR): In 2008, our county was declared a federal disaster area eight times.

Beth Ingram (BI): As vice president of the Arkansas Hospital Association, I have a different perspective on the disasters that have hit our state and our hospitals. Hospitals are the lifeline and refuge for the community and the place everyone turns to for shelter, food, and patient care. At the Arkansas Hospital Association, the community expects our lights to always be on, that we always have electricity, and the community knows we will take them in, no matter what.

Interviewer: Please describe the disasters in question.

ALR: On Monday evening January 26, 2009, the counties of north central Arkansas began seeing dropping temperatures with rain in the forecast. By 12:00 am on Tuesday morning we began to see freezing rain, and by the time I left for work that morning we had a continuous flow of heavy freezing rain. The trees and power lines were already heavy under the weight of the ice, power was out in several areas, and telephone lines were out. On Tuesday evening we lost cell service in the area, and the generator to Calico Rock's water supply went out, leaving the town without water. Without traditional communication, it seemed that everyone around the world knew what we were going through but us. The hospital staff (at both facilities) continued doing what they do best, taking care of patients. Patient care went on amidst intermittent generator power, no standard communication lines, leaking roofs, increased patient volumes, low supplies, low staffing because of hazardous roads, and no water in Calico Rock.

KR: On February 5th, 2008, an F4 tornado came through our town of 2,500 people, missing the hospital but destroying many homes and killing one person and injuring many. We were without power for a couple of days and parts of the county went two weeks before power was restored. The tornado stayed on the ground for 123 miles. Our hospital implemented our disaster plan and worked all night long treating, admitting, and transferring patients. We served as an emergency shelter for many that first night, mainly for those whose homes had been destroyed. We served soup and sandwiches until we ran out of food. People brought their pets with them. Our lobbies and hallways were full of families sleeping and huddled together. The tornado destroyed a home for the disabled, and their residents wandered into our facility for hours. The neighboring towns and the Arkansas Department of Emergency Management (ADEM) were of great assistance. FEMA came and stayed for several weeks and served us very well.

Interviewer: Prior to these events, had your facility prepared by conducting drills and exercises?

BI: All hospitals in Arkansas are partners in preparedness efforts for the entire state. Each hospital belongs to a regional group that regularly meets, educates, and conducts drills. With preparedness dollars brought into our state by the Office of the Assistant Secretary for Preparedness and Response (ASPR) funds, hospitals are very well prepared with equipment, training, communications tools, pharmaceuticals, and supplies to meet any type of disaster. Because the regional groups hold periodic (most of them meet monthly) meetings, they have formed bonds with their neighboring hospitals, county emergency operations centers (EOCs), the Arkansas Department of Emergency Management, and the state Department of Health. Through these bonds they know that they are never alone in a time of disaster. On a scale of 1 to 10, I would say our hospitals would rate about an 8 in disaster preparedness, because there is always room for improvement and continued growth and development.

KR: We had both tabletop drills and exercises prior to the tornado event and they served us well. Communication was tenuous at best and impossible at times. Local law enforcement gave us great support, and within several hours the National Guard arrived to secure destroyed homes and businesses. The communication networks set up by the state and ADEM were up but not functional as there were no directories, and despite good efforts, they were not able to facilitate evacuation of patients. Communication was done the old-fashioned way, based on personal relationships between some of our staff and staff at the medical centers. A staff recall was not needed, as virtually the entire staff returned to the facility before a recall could be activated.

Interviewer: Did the ownership/corporate structure of your hospital affect your response to this event?

ALR: Yes. I was able to see the event from the perspective of a county-owned facility (FCH) and a private facility (CMC). Fulton County officials took very good care of FCH during this disaster. They provided fuel, ice removal, support, and even a backup generator when one of the FCH generators began to struggle. Although the city officials of Calico Rock, our physicians, and our staff prepared early for the storm and came together to continue to take care of patients on generator power and a manual water supply, they did not have the immediate access to help that FCH had.

Interviewer: Do you feel you had the right culture to sustain you through this disaster? If so, describe the characteristics of your culture. If not, why and how would you or how have you changed the culture for future disaster response?

ALR: The cultures at both hospitals are different, but I would say they both had the strong teamwork necessary to sustain them. Although FCH had the strongest county governance support, CMC had the strongest culture and a natural calmness that was easily passed along to patients who looked to the hospital as a safety net. On Thursday afternoon, with still no word from the electricity supplier as to when the hospital would have power or water, I went to Dr. Meryl Grasse's house to give him an update. Dr. Grasse is the original founder of CMC and is currently the medical director. He has been the strong stable force of CMC for over 50 years and is the greatest man I have ever known. I found him and his wife, Gladys, at home enjoying a fire, and they invited me to sit with them and have tea and pretzels. The calming nature that Dr. Grasse has passed on to the physicians and staff of CMC for the last 50 years was evident in this disaster as well.

KR: We are a very rural facility in a sparsely populated, geographically mountainous, and dispersed region. The workforce is cohesive with a sense of obligation and responsibility to the organization, the greater community, and to each other. They came with overnight bags to stay for the long haul. We had trouble getting key staff to go home or to bed so they would be rested to cover the next several days of disaster staffing.

BI: I definitely think Arkansas hospitals have the right culture to sustain them through any disaster. We simply help each other: This may mean that a community volunteer at the hospital provides food and clothing for disaster victims or that a hospital helps caregivers in another state care for patients when they are dealing with a disastrous hurricane and its aftermath.

Interviewer: How did you communicate internally and externally during this disaster?

ALR: The Arkansas Wireless Information Network (AWIN) radio was our only means of communication during the ice storm.

BI: Arkansas hospitals, through preparedness funds, are equipped with 800 MHz radios, ham radios and improved towers (including training for the radio operators), and other redundant communication methods. In the Little Rock area, the metropolitan hospital disaster group purchased a "hotline" phone that is installed in each hospital emergency department (ED). When an emergency arises at one hospital (or in the community), one person picks up the "red" phone and it automatically rings down through the line until everyone has picked up to receive the message. The group has had several occasions to use the phones and the system works very well.

Interviewer: What was the biggest challenge to your employees and your medical staff during this disaster?

ALR: Communication. AWIN communications were our lifeline during this disaster due to an extended outage affecting landline, cellular, and Internet communications. Many of our staff needed to be trained to use the AWIN, specifically how to navigate the different MAC channels. Reception was a problem at CMC and in most areas. At FCH, the AWIN worked in the ED, but reception was limited.

KR: Our greatest challenge was not knowing what was going on outside the hospital, as all of our employees had friends and families that were lost or out of contact. The evacuation of neurosurgery patients was particularly difficult as this state has a recognized shortage of specialists in neurosurgery.

BI: The biggest challenge during the ice storms was that employees' and physicians' homes were without power, so while they were helping out at the hospital (which was most likely on generator power), they had families and pets at home without power. There is also always the problem of "caring for the caregiver." Hospital staff tend to go the extra mile without regard to their personal well-being. They go through a disaster without thinking about a clock or food or personal hygiene. Often when the crisis is over, they collapse or become ill. We have done some training for hospital staff this past year on caring for themselves and their coworkers during and after a disaster.

Interviewer: What agencies, individuals, or organizations were most helpful? Did any impede your ability to respond?

ALR: The Arkansas Department of Health was extremely helpful in getting the energy supplier Entergy to respond to CMC and Calico Rock's need for power. Ozark Health Hospital in Clinton, Arkansas, was extremely helpful at staying on the AWIN radio and making phone calls for us.

KR: The local law enforcement agencies, Arkansas Department of Health, and state and county emergency management departments were all very helpful.

BI: The Arkansas Department of Health operates an EOC that activates immediately when a disaster occurs anywhere in the state. The staff and crew are exceptional at what they do. The Arkansas Department of Emergency Management is always there and hospitals work well with that organization.

Interviewer: What do you wish you had known before this event?

ALR: Everyone needed to have been trained on the AWIN radio. We had limited staff at both facilities that understood how to operate the radio.

BI: Much more should have been known about how the various federal, state, and local government entities work. We learned that county emergency officials are the key contact and very, very important in ensuring that the proper government entities respond to your area. However, in Arkansas, many of these officials are part-time and seem to have little oversight.

Interviewer: What did you do that you feel was right?

ALR: Healthcare workers do so many things "right" on a daily basis, but to see the teamwork between the community, physicians, and staff and their total commitment to providing quality patient care during a difficult time makes healthcare a wonderful mission. My challenge was to keep the mood positive, continue to build morale, and create community.

BI: It goes back to hospitals helping each other. We can make all these disaster or emergency plans, but when something terrible happens to one of our own, things just fall into place. No Arkansas hospital should ever feel alone. There's always someone calling or driving through rain, ice, and floods to see about supplies, food, and repairs.

Interviewer: What would you do differently? How has the hospital changed after this event?

ALR: There are several things we are doing differently or that we have learned:

◆ We will keep the diesel tank used to fuel our generator full during the winter months to offset the chance of unexpected weather.

- We now have emergency contacts established for when we have extended periods of need (such as agreements between the county, prison, and school system).
- We have put together emergency kits that include items such as flashlights, battery-operated radios, and extra batteries.
- We have more portable radios that we can leave in different areas and that are within range of the local fire station.
- In-service training has been conducted on the AWIN radio to make it more useful. A manual has been developed to guide employees through the process.
- We know that we can have the prison do laundry and the fire department will assist with portable water.
- We know that we can get food and pharmacy supplies from the local grocery, pharmacies, and neighboring hospitals.

The ice storm provided a great learning experience and did showcase how well department managers could function in crisis.

KR: I would have trained several of our staff to become shortwave radio operators.

Interviewer: Were there any unintended consequences of this experience?

BI: In each disaster, we learn just how much the hospital means to the community. You don't hear that on a day-to-day basis, but it comes home during a disaster.

Interviewer: What surprised or shocked you about your experience?

ALR: I was struck by the overwhelming calmness of the staff at CMC. If anyone arrived during the time immediately after the storm (ignoring the hanging ice, broken tree limbs, and the electric entrance doors hanging ajar), they walked inside to a sense of "business as usual."

KR: I was surprised by the number of children that were injured by the tornado. The day was warm for February and the tornado hit at approximately 5:30 pm, and many children were playing outside. We treated a lot of cuts and abrasions from flying debris. The power and energy of the storm was stunning. It was a mile wide at the base and moved at 70 miles per hour. If you were in its path, you were in trouble. A lot of storm shelters were installed after this storm.

Interviewer: What advice would you give for those who will face similar situations in the future?

ALR: Train and exercise, train and exercise, train and exercise. Especially train everyone on your radio system, because you never know who will need to know how to operate it. Also, get to know your emergency managers and make them your best friends.

Interviewer: What did you learn about yourself, your team, and your facility?

ALR: I learned that mission outweighs consequences. Many of our employees chose healthcare careers to comfort, heal, and improve health, and this is what they did in spite of the difficult circumstances that surrounded them at work and at home. Most of our employees live in the country and they were the last ones to get power restored. Many went up to three weeks without power or water.

Interviewer: What upcoming likely events have you prepared for?

ALR: We are currently preparing for influenza and a potential H1N1 pandemic.

KR: We are preparing for the H1N1 pandemic, chemical spills, and terrorist events.

BI: A tornado destroying a hospital, chemical spills, school bus wrecks in a town with only one very small hospital, and earthquakes.

Interviewer: What have you done specifically to prepare your facility for likely events?

ALR: We actively participate in our region's disaster preparedness committee, are training in emergency response and management, and are conducting routine and annual exercises.

Interviewer: What are the most important leadership characteristics that helped you to prepare for and respond to this event?

ALR: One of the most important leadership characteristics that helped me prepare for and respond to this disaster was my organizational skills. In strategic planning, we worked diligently to develop a strong, clearly defined organizational chart and empower the employees. This structure gave the staff confidence, comfort, and a good understanding of their roles and responsibilities. With many managers, directors, and administration unable to get to the hospital, it was fortunate that the employees were capable to manage the response.

KR: Don't panic and don't get angry; everyone is already on edge. Work hard to determine the facts of your particular event and keep everyone informed as the disaster unfolds. Be visible and visit the treatment areas where the clinical work is being done. Nothing beats seeing it for yourself, and the staff appreciates your presence. Keep the media informed and help them to the greatest extent possible because they will be writing a story whether you like it or not. You should also help the staff find out about their families and provide childcare if necessary.

BI: The most important leadership characteristics are the ability to know the right contacts during an event, to know who is in charge, and to be able to direct staff appropriately.

Interviewer: What were the personal consequences for you or your leadership staff from responding to this event?

ALR: I feel that we all came through the storm feeling closer to our staff and peers while feeling more like family than coworkers. Our showers became community showers with a waiting line in the mornings. Clothes that looked like they matched in the dark early morning often didn't match when you arrived at work. So, we learned how to laugh when sometimes life just wasn't that funny. In the words of Stan Toler, "Humor is to life what shock absorbers are to automobiles."

References

About.com. 2010. "Disaster Recovery Decision Making for Small Business." [Online information; retrieved 10/01/2010.] http://sbinformation.about. com/od/disastermanagement/a/disasterrecover.htm.

Aguirre, B. E. 2006. "On the Concept of Resilience." Preliminary paper. Newark, DE: Disaster Research Center, University of Delaware.

American College of Healthcare Executives (ACHE). 2009. "Healthcare Executives' Role in Emergency Preparedness." Policy statement. [Online document; retrieved 7/29/10.] www.ache.org/policy/emergency_preparedness.cfm.

American Heritage Dictionary of the English Language, 4th ed. 2006. Boston: Houghton Mifflin Harcourt.

American Hospital Association (AHA). 2009. *AHA 2009 Environmental Scan*. Chicago: American Hospital Association.

Ames, S., training and exercise coordinator, Oklahoma State Department of Health, Oklahoma City, OK, personal correspondence.

Associated Press. 2005. "Too Many People in Nature's Way." [Online information; retrieved 9/6/05.] www.wired.com/news/culture/1,68756-0.html.

Auf der Heide, E. 1996. "Disaster Planning, Part II: Disaster Problems, Issues, and Challenges Identified in the Research Literature." *Emergency Medicine Clinics of North America* 14 (2): 453–80.

———. 1989. *Disaster Response: Principles of Preparation and Coordination*. [Online book; retrieved 7/29/10.] http://orgmail2.coe-dmha.org/dr/flash.htm.

Barbera, J. A., D. J. Yeatts, and A. G. MacIntyre. 2009. "Challenge of Hospital Emergency Preparedness: Analysis and Recommendations." *Disaster Medicine and Public Health Preparedness* 3 (Suppl. 1): S74–S79.

Barbisch, D. F., and K. L. Koenig. 2006. "Understanding Surge Capacity: Essential Elements." *Academic Emergency Medicine* 13 (11): 1098-102.

Baum, N., and J. W. McDaniel. 2008. *Disaster Planning for the Clinical Practice.* Sudbury, MA: Jones and Bartlett.

Bednarz, D., and K. Bradford. 2008. "Medicine at the Crossroads of Energy and Climate Change." [Online information; retrieved 7/26/10.] www.energybulletin.net/node/38642#sdendnote13sym.

Bell, J. R., and S. Borenstein. 2010. "2010's World Gone Wild: Quakes, Floods, Blizzards." [online article; accessed 1/3/11] http://www.msnbc.msn.com/id/40739667/ns/us_news-2010_year_in_review/

Boatright, C., and K. J. McGlown. 2005. "Homeland Security Challenges in Nursing Practice." *Nursing Clinics of North America* 40 (3): 481–97.

Bruneau, M., S. E. Chang, R. Equchi, G. C. Lee, T. D. O'Rourke, A. M. Reinhorn, M. Shinozuka, K. Tierney, W. A. Wallace, and D. von Winterfeldt. 2003. "A Framework to Quantitatively Assess and Enhance the Seismic Resilience of Communities." *Earthquake Spectra* 19 (4): 733–52.

Bruntland, G. H. 2003. "Health Disaster Management: Guidelines for Evaluation and Research in the Utstein Style." Foreword. *Prehospital and Disaster Medicine* 17 (Suppl. 3): 1–24.

Bullock, J., and G. Haddow. 2006. *Introduction to Homeland Security,* 2nd ed. Amsterdam: Butterworth-Heinemann.

Bush, G. W. 2003. Homeland Security Presidential Directive/HSPD-5. [Online document; retrieved 7/9/10.] www.vet.utk.edu/cafsp/resources/pdf/Homeland%20Security%20Presidential%20Directives%205,%207,%208,%20&%209.pdf.

CBS Chicago. 2010. "Experts Warn of Future Chicago Water Shortage." [Online information; retrieved 7/26/10.] http://cbs2chicago.com/local/chicago.water.shortage.2.1649418.html.

Center for Biosecurity of UPMC. 2009. *Hospitals Rising to the Challenge: The First Five Years of the U.S. Hospital Preparedness Program and Priorities Going Forward.* [Online evaluation report; retrieved 6/29/10.] www.upmc-biosecurity.org/website/resources/publications/2009/pdf/2009-04-16-hppreport.pdf.

Centers for Disease Control and Prevention. n.d. "Questions and Answers About Avian Influenza (Bird Flu) and Avian Influenza A (H5N1) Virus." [Online information; retrieved 7/26/10.] www.cdc.gov/flu/avian/gen-info/qa.htm.

Centre for Research on the Epidemiology of Disasters (CRED). 2008. Brussels, Belgium: CRED.

Chaffee, M. 2009. "Willingness of Health Care Personnel to Work in a Disaster: An Integrative Review of the Literature." *Disaster Medicine and Public Health Preparedness* 3: 42–56.

Climate Services and Monitoring Division, NOAA/National Climatic Data Center (NOAA/NCDC). 2010. "U.S. Tornado Climatology." Overview. [Online information, retrieved 12/7/10.] www.ncdc.noaa.gov/oa/climate/severeweather/tornadoes.html.

Digital Journal. 2010. "Climate Change and the 'Wacky Weather' of Oregon, Louisiana." [Online information; retrieved 7/26/10.] www.digitaljournal. com/article/287628.

Dror, Y. 1988. "Decision Making Under Disaster Conditions." In L. K. Comfort, *Managing Disaster: Strategies and Policy Perspectives,* 255–75. Durham, NC: Duke University Press.

Dunham, W. 2009. "Antarctic Ice Sheet Collapse May Swamp U.S. Coasts." Reuters. [Online information; retrieved 7/26/10.] www.reuters.com/article/ idUSTRE51472Q20090205?feedType=RSS&feedName=environmentNews.

Faust, E. 2009. "Climate and Climate Change: Data, Facts, Background." In *Topics Geo: Natural Catastrophes 2009. Analyses, Assessments, Positions.* [Online publication; retrieved 12/13/10.] www.preventionweb.net/ files/13196_topics2009.pdf.

Federal Emergency Management Agency (FEMA). 2010a. "Declared Disasters by Year or State." [Online information; retrieved 6/28/10.] www.fema.gov/ news/disaster_totals_annual.fema.

———. 2010b. "NIMS Resource Center: Glossary." [Online information; retrieved 6/28/10.] www.fema.gov/emergency/nims/Glossary.shtm

———. 2010c. "Are You Ready?" [online information; accessed 2/9/11] www. fema.gov/areyouready/flood.shtm

———. 2008. "Catastrophic Incident Annex," 4. [Online information; retrieved 12/13/10.] www.fema.gov/pdf/emergency/nrf/nrf_ CatastrophicIncidentAnnex.pdf.

———. 2006. "NIMS Implementation Activities for Hospitals and Healthcare Systems." [Online document; retrieved 7/9/10.] www.fema.gov/pdf/emergency/nims/imp_act_hos_hlth.pdf.

Fink, S. 1986. *Crisis Management: Planning for the Inevitable.* New York: Amacom.

Flynn, S. 2007. *The Edge of Disaster: Rebuilding a Resilient Nation.* New York: Random House.

Gartner, Inc. 2001. "Disaster Recovery Plans and Systems Are Essential." [Online information retrieved 12/7/10.] www.gartner.com/DisplayDocument?id=340749&acsFlg=accessBought.

Gilbert, M. E. 1982. "Management of a Crisis." *Bulletin*, U.S. Coast Guard Commandant [now *Coast Guard Magazine*] (November/December).

Glantz, M. H., and Q. Ye. 2010. *Usable Thoughts: Climate, Water and Weather in the Twenty-first Century.* New York: United Nations University Press.

Godschalk, D. R. 2003. "Urban Hazard Mitigation: Creating Resilient Cities." *Natural Hazards Review* 4 (3): 136–43.

Greater New York Hospital Association (GNYHA). 2006. "Bulletin: Recovery Checklist for Hospitals After a Disaster." [Online document; retrieved 8/25/10.] www.nyc.gov/html/doh/downloads/pdf/bhpp/bhpp-hospital-tools-checklist.pdf.

Gupta, S. 2010. "Swine Flu Vaccine Tossed." CNN Health, The Chart. [Online information; retrieved 7/26/10.] http://pagingdrgupta.blogs.cnn.com/2010/07/01/swine-flu-vaccine-tossed/.

Harrald, J. R. 1998. "Linking Corporate Crisis Management to Natural Disaster Reduction." Washington, DC: Institute for Crisis, Disaster, and Risk Management, George Washington University.

Heath, R. 1997. "Dealing with the Complete Crisis: Management Shell Structure." Contribution to the 1997 International Emergency Management Society Conference. Roskilde, Denmark: Riso National Lab.

Hess, C. M. 2004. "Going from a 'Federal' to a 'National' Approach: The Interim National Response Plan, and the National Incident Management System." EIIP Virtual Forum presentation. January 14.

Himalayan Times. 2010. "Water Shortage Hits Rukum Hospital." [Online information; retrieved 7/26/10.] www.thehimalayantimes.com/fullNews.php?headline=Water+shortage+hits+Rukum+hospital+&NewsID=250678.

HP and SCORE: Counselors to America's Small Business. 2007. "Impact on U.S. Small Business from Natural & Man-Made Disasters." [Online information, retrieved 12/9/10]. www.edwardsinformation.com/content/ImpactofDisaster.pdf.

IBM. 2010. "Business Continuity Planning." [Online information; retrieved 8/3/10.] www-03.ibm.com/systems/business_resiliency/continuity_planning/.

Ikinci, S. 2007. "Serious Water Shortage in Turkey." World Socialist Web Site. [Online information; retrieved 7/26/10.] www.wsws.org/articles/2007/aug2007/anka-a22.shtml.

Institute of Medicine (IOM). 2009. *Guidance for Establishing Crisis Standards of Care for Use in Disaster Situations: A Letter Report.* Washington, DC: National Academies Press.

Insurance Information Institute. 2010. "Catastrophes: U.S." [Online information; retrieved 6/29/10.] www.iii.org/media/facts/statsbyissue/catastrophes.

Insurance Information Network of California (IINC). 2006. "Are You Financially Prepared for an Earthquake?" [Online information, retrieved 12/9/10.] www.iinc.org/articles/29/1/Are-You-Financially-Prepared-for-an-Earthquake/Page1.html.

Insurance Services Office. 2010. "PCS Catastrophe Serial Numbers." Property Claim Services. [Online information; retrieved 11/15/10.] www.iso.com/Products/Property-Claim-Services/PCS-Catastrophe-Serial-Numbers.html.

Insure.com. 2009. "The Basics of Earthquake Insurance." [Online information; retrieved 12/9/10.] www.insure.com/articles/homeinsurance/quake.html.

Interagency Working Group on Climate Change and Health. 2008. *A Human Health Perspective on Climate Change: A Report Outlining the Research Needs on the Human Health Effects of Climate Change.* [Online information; retrieved 7/26/10.] www.cdc.gov/climatechange/pubs/HHCC_Final_508.pdf.

Kraft, M. B. 2010. "Bioterrorism Threats Highlighted in Hearing." [Online information; retrieved 7/26/10.] http://counterterrorismblog.org/2010/03/bioterrorism_threats_highlight.php.

Landeman, L. Y. 2005. *Public Health Management of Disasters. The Practice Guide,* 2nd ed. New York: American Public Health Association.

Landsea, C. 2010. "Subject: E19) How Many Direct Hits by Hurricanes of Various Categories Have Affected Each State?" [Online information, retrieved 12/7/10]. www.aoml.noaa.gov/hrd/tcfaq/E19.html.

Lemonick, M. 2010. "The Secret of Sea Level Rise: It Will Vary Greatly by Region." [Online information; retrieved 7/26/10.] http://e360.yale.edu/content/feature.msp?id=2255.

Mileti, D. S. 1999. *Disasters by Design: A Reassessment of Natural Hazards in the United States.* Washington, DC: Joseph Henry Press.

Mitroff, I. I. 2001. *Managing Crises Before They Happen: What Every Executive and Manager Needs to Know About Crisis Management.* New York: Amaco.

Mitroff, I. I., and T. C. Pomchant. 1992. *Transforming the Crisis-Prone Organization.* San Francisco: Jossey-Bass.

MSNBC.com. 2010. "Jan.-June Warmest First Half of Year on Record." [Online information; retrieved 7/26/10.] www.msnbc.msn.com/id/38263788/.

Multihazard Mitigation Council, National Institute of Building Sciences. 2005. "Natural Hazard Mitigation Saves: An Independent Study to Assess the Future Savings from Mitigation Activities." [Online document; retrieved 8/24/10.] www.nibs.org/index.php/mmc/projects/nhms.

Munich Re. 2010a. "NatCatSERVICE." [Online information; retrieved 6/29/10.] www.munichre.com/en/reinsurance/business/non-life/georisks/ natcatservice/annual_statistics/default.aspx.

————. 2010b. *Topics GEO: Natural Catastrophes 2009. Analysis, Assessments, Positions.* [Online publication; retrieved 6/29/10.] www.preventionweb.net/ files/13196_topics2009.pdf.

National Academies Press (NAP). 2010. "Review of the U.S. Geological Survey's Volcano Hazards Program (2000)." [Online information, retrieved 12/7/10]. www.nap.edu/openbook.php?record_id=9884&page=15.

National Fire Protection Association (NFPA). 2004. *NFPA 1600 Standard on Disaster/ Emergency Management and Business Continuity Program.* Quincy, MA: NFPA.

National Institute of Allergy and Infectious Diseases. n.d. "Emerging and Re-emerging Infectious Diseases." [Online information; retrieved 7/26/10.] www.niaid.nih.gov/topics/emerging/Pages/Default.aspx.

National Oceanic and Atmospheric Administration (NOAA). 2010. "Past Tracks of Landfalling United States Major Hurricanes." National Hurricane Center, National Weather Service. [Online information; retrieved 6/28/10.] www. nhc.noaa.gov/pastall.shtml#tracks_us.

————. 2006. "NOAA Reviews Record-Setting 2005 Atlantic Hurricane Season: Active Hurricane Era Likely to Continue." [Online article; retrieved 6/28/10.] www.noaanews.noaa.gov/stories2005/s2540.htm.

National Resources Defense Council. 2010."Climate Change, Water, and Risk: Current Water Demands Are Not Sustainable." [Online information; retrieved 7/26/10.] www.nrdc.org/globalWarming/watersustainability/files/WaterRisk.pdf.

National Science and Technology Council. 2003. "Reducing Disaster Vulnerability Through Science and Technology." [Online information, retrieved 12/9/10.] www.unisdr.org/eng/mdgs-drr/national-reports/U-S-report.pdf.

Neck, C. P., and C. C. Manz. 1994. "From GroupThink to Teamthink: Toward the Creation of Constructive Thought Patterns in Self-Managing Work Teams." *Human Relations* 457 (8): 922–52.

New York Times. n.d. "Health Guide: Avian Influenza." [Online information; retrieved 7/26/10.] http://health.nytimes.com/health/guides/disease/avian-influenza/overview.html.

9/11 Commission. 2004. *The 9/11 Commission Report.* Washington, DC: U.S. Government Printing Office.

Njeru, G. 2010. "Kenya: Climate Change Water Crisis Impacts Hospital Maternal Care." [Online information; retrieved 7/26/10.] http://women-newsnetwork.net/2010/07/13/kenyamaternalh2o.

Northeast States Emergency Consortium (NESEC). n.d. "Fires: Did You Know?" [Online information, retrieved 12/9/10.] www.nesec.org/hazards/fires.cfm.

Oklahoma Legislature. 2003. Catastrophic Health Emergency Powers Act, c. 473, SS1.

Organisation for Economic Co-operation and Development. 2007. "Climate Change Could Triple Population at Risk for Coastal Flooding by 2070, Finds OEC." [Online information; retrieved 11/16/2010.] http://www.oecd.org/document/4/0,3343,en_2649_201185_39727650_1_1_1_1,00.html.

Pine, J. C. 2009. "Session 5: Political and Legal Issues." In *Catastrophe Readiness and Response.* [Online PowerPoint slide presentation; retrieved 8/4/10.] http://training.fema.gov/EMIWeb/edu/crr.asp.

Post, J. M. 1993. "The Impact of Crisis-Induced Stress on Policy Makers." In *Avoiding Inadvertent War*, edited by A. George. Boulder, CO: Westview Press.

Qureshi, K., R. R. Gershon, M. F. Sherman, T. Straub, E. Gebbie, M. McCollum, M. J. Erwin, and S. S. Morse. 2005. "Health Care Workers' Ability and Willingness to Report to Duty During Catastrophic Disasters." *Journal of Urban Health* 82 (3): 378–88.

RAND Corporation. 2006. "RAND Study Estimates New Orleans Population to Climb to About 272,000 in 2008." [Online article; retrieved 9/5/09.] www.rand.org/news/press.06.03.15.html.

Ray, J. 2009. "Federal Declaration of a Public Health Emergency." *Biosecurity and Bioterrorism: Biodefense Strategy, Practice, and Service* 7 (3): 251–58.

Reilly, A. H. 1993. "Preparing for the Worst: The Process of Effective Crisis Management." *Industrial and Environmental Quarterly* 7 (2): 118.

Ruback, J., S. Wells, and R. Bissell. 2009. "New Methods of Planning for Catastrophic Disasters." Instructor notes for session 12. Baltimore, MD: University of Baltimore.

Schmid, R. E. 2006. "Melting Ice Raises Sea Level, Journal Says." *Birmingham News,* March 24, 6A.

Shaw, G. L. 2006. "Business Crisis in Continuity Management." In *Disciplines, Disasters, and Emergency Management: The Convergence and Divergence of Concepts, Issues and Trends from the Research Literature,* edited by D. A. McIntire. Washington, DC: Federal Emergency Management Agency.

Shaw, G. L., and J. R. Harrald. 2004. "Identification of the Core Competencies Required of Executive Level Business Crisis and Continuity Managers." *Journal of Homeland Security and Emergency Management* 1 (1).

Steinberg, A., and R. F. Ritzmann. 1990. "A Living Systems Approach to Understanding the Concept of Stress." *Behavioral Sciences* 35 (2): 138–46.

Stone, B. 2010. "Heat Waves on the Rise in Big Cities." [Online information; retrieved 7/26/10.] www.cnn.com/2010/OPINION/07/07/stone.city.heat. wave/index.html.

Sundnes, K. O., and M. L. Birnbaum. 2003. "Health Disaster Management: Guidelines for Evaluation and Research in the Utstein Style." *Prehospital and Disaster Medicine* 17 (Suppl. 3): 1–24.

2030 Research Center. 2007. "Nation Under Siege." [Online information; retrieved 7/26/10.] http://solveclimate.com/resource/nation-under-siege.

United Nations Environment Programme (UNEP). 2006. *Planet in Peril: Atlas of Current Threats to People and the Environment.* Norway: UNEP/GRID-Arendal.

University of Pittsburgh Medical Center (UPMC) Center for Biosecurity. 2010a. "How to Lead During Bioattacks with the Public's Trust and Help: A Manual for Mayors, Governors, and Top Health Officials." [Online information; retrieved 5/21/10.] www.upmc-biosecurity.org/website/resources/leadership/.

———. 2010b. "The Next Challenge in Healthcare Preparedness: Catastrophic Health Events." [Online information; retrieved 12/8/10.] www.upmc-biosecurity.org/website/resources/publications/2010/pdf/2010-01-29-prepreport.pdf.

U.S. Department of Homeland Security (DHS). 2008. *National Response Framework.* Washington, DC: Federal Emergency Management Agency.

———. 2007. "Homeland Security Presidential Directive 21: Public Health and Medical Preparedness." [Online document; retrieved 7/21/10.] www.dhs.gov/xabout/laws/gc_1219263961449.shtm#1.

———. 2004. *National Response Plan (NRP)*. Final Draft. Washington DC: DHS.

———. 2003. "Homeland Security Directive 8: National Preparedness." [Online information; retrieved 7/9/10.] www.dhs.gov/xabout/laws/gc_1215444247124.shtm.

U.S. Geological Survey (USGS). 2010. "USGS Natural Hazards Programs: Lessons Learned for Reducing Risk." [Online information; retrieved 12/7/10.] http://water.usgs.gov/wid/html/HRDS.html.

U.S. Geological Survey Earthquake Hazards Program. 2009. "Top Earthquake States." [Online information; retrieved 3/18/09.] http://earthquake.usgs.gov/regional/states/top_states.php.

U.S. Geological Survey Landslide Hazards Program. 2009. "Landslides 101: Where do Landslides Occur?" [Online information; retrieved 12/9/10.] http://landslides.usgs.gov/learning/ls101.php.

Veenema, T. G. 2003. "Essentials of Disaster Planning." *Disaster Nursing and Emergency Preparedness for Chemical, Biological, and Radiological Terrorism and Other Hazards*, edited by T. G. Veenema, 3–19. New York: Springer.

VOANews.com. 2010. "Water Shortages Continue to Threaten the World's Growing Population." [Online information; retrieved 7/26/10.] www1.voanews.com/learningenglish/home/Water-Shortages-89876647.html.

Watkins, M. D., and M. H. Bazerman. 2003. *Predictable Surprises: The Disasters You Should Have Seen Coming*. Cambridge, MA: Harvard Business School Publishing.

Weyerhaueser. 2005. *Hurricane Katrina: Rebuilding a Community. An Employer's Guide to Assisting Employees.* [Online document; retrieved 8/25/10.] www.weyerhaeuser.com/pdfs/sustainability/HurricaneKatrinaResponse-EmployersGuide.pdf.

White House. 2003. "National Strategy for the Physical Protection of Critical Infrastructure and Key Assets." Washington DC: White House.

Wirtz, A. 2010. "Great Natural Catastrophes—Causes and Effects." In *Topics Geo: Natural Catastrophes 2009. Analysis, Assessments, Positions,* edited by Munich Re, 35–37. [Online publication; retrieved 12/13/10.] www.preventionweb.net/files/13196_topics2009.pdf.

Woodworth, B. H. 2007. "The Key Elements of Business Resiliency Success." [Online information; retrieved 12/8/10.] www.govtech.com/public-safety/5-Disaster-Response-Tips.html.

World Commission on Environment and Development. 1987. *Our Common Future*. London: Oxford University Press.

World Health Organization. 2010. "Global Alert and Response (GAR): Avian Influenza." [Online information; retrieved 7/26/10.] www.who.int/csr/disease/avian_influenza/en.

Wright, J. E. 1976. "Interorganizational Systems and Networks in Mass Casualty Situations." In *Disaster Planning, Part II: Disaster Problems, Issues, and Challenges Identified in the Research Literature*, edited by E. Auf der Heide, 453–74.

Zinkewicz, P. 2005. "Business Interruption Insurance—Death Protection for a Business." [Online article; retrieved 6/29/10.] http://findarticles.com/p/articles/mi_qa3615/is_200507/ai_n14775710.

Index

Enterprise management, 55

Environmental sustainability, 92

Epidemics, 137; crisis standards of care for, 46–47

Equipment: disaster-related damage to, 123–124; valuation for insurance coverage, 105

Ethics, in healthcare management, 37–38

Europe: avian influenza (H5N1) in, 136–137; natural catastrophes in, 13

Evacuations, 40; FEMA reimbursement for, 127–128; FEMA system for, 80; mass, 32, 40; of patients, 74–75, 80, 127–128

Event, *versus* incident, 17–18

Exercises, 56, 147–151, 162, 163; budget for, 100, 101; CEOs' knowledge of, 60–61; ethical issues in, 38

Expenses, disaster-related increase in, 101–103

External collaboration, in emergency preparedness, 54–59

External recovery, 93–95

Family: of hospital staff, 75, 77, 81, 82, 177; of mass casualty victims, 85

Fatalities, disaster-related, 8, 9, 18

Fatigue, avoidance of, 82–83

Federal agencies. *See also names of specific agencies:* regulatory and standard-setting, 33–35

Federal declarations of disaster, 7, 8, 24, 25, 26, 94

Federal Emergency Management Agency (FEMA), 9, 21, 174; all-hazards planning approach of, 42; debris removal assistance from, 122; disaster assistance policy of, 125–129;

disaster recovery resources of, 94, 95, 98; federal declarations of disaster and, 130; filing of claims with, 102, 115–116, 120–122; free emergency training courses of, 60; grants and reimbursements from, 125–129; hazard mitigation expenditures by, 96; *Helping Children Cope with a Disaster,* 96–97; hospital evacuation reimbursement by, 127–128; hospital evacuation system of, 80; Incident Management Systems Division, 34; Individuals and Households Program of, 94; *NIMS Implementation Activities for Hospitals and Healthcare Systems,* 29–31; Public Assistance Program of, 94–95; unreliability of, 69

Federal government. *See also specific federal agencies:* catastrophic incident response process of, 34–35; disaster recovery resources of, 94–95, 130; national response doctrine of, 20–21; response to multiple or successive catastrophic incidents, 42; role in disaster preparedness, 19; role in emergency response, 24

FEMA. *See* Federal Emergency Management Agency (FEMA)

Financial actions, during and after catastrophic events, 119–130; applying for payer advances, 120; checklist of, 119; filing of insurance and FEMA claims, 120–125; use of line of credit, 120; working with bond trustees, 129; working with credit enhancement firms, 129

Financial planning activities, for catastrophic events, 99–118; for aftereffects of disasters, 117, 118; arranging

U.S. Department of Health and Human Services: Assistant Secretary for Preparedness and Response (ASPR) of, 25, 31, 34; Secretary of, 25, 26

U.S. Department of Homeland Security: definition of incidents, 17; disaster recovery resources of, 98; National Planning Scenarios of, 16; National Preparedness Guidelines of, 27, 29; National Preparedness Strategy of, 27–28; Secretary of, 28

U.S. Department of Labor, 93

United Way, 116

University of Pittsburgh Medical Center (UPMC), 59; Center for Biosecurity, 46–47

University of Texas Health Sciences Center, Houston, Texas, 153–154

University of Texas Medical Branch, Galveston, Texas, 153–169

Vaccinations, 87, 136

Veterans Administration, Nine Step Emergency Management Planning Process of, 43–45

Vietnam, avian influenza (H5N1) in, 136

Volcanoes, 3

Voluntary Organizations Active in Disaster (VOAD), 94

Vulnerability: to disasters, 10; of special needs populations, 37–38

Wallace, Mark, 167, 171

Washington, D.C., effect of sea-level rise on, 133, 134

Water shortage, global risk of, 134–135

Water supply, disaster-related loss of, 112, 173, 174, 175

Weapons of mass destruction (WMD), 39, 40

Wildfires, 3, 13, 57

Woodworth, Brent H., 50

World Commission on Environment and Development, Brundtland Commission of, 92

World Health Organization (WHO), 134–135, 137

World Meteorological Organization, 132

"Worst Case Scenario" game, 37

Wright, Randall, 165–172

Acknowledgments

While the authors' names may be the ones on the cover of this book, putting together a work like this requires a lot of hard work from a team of dedicated professionals. We wish to thank Eileen Lynch, our editor at Health Administration Press, for her patience and creativity in delivering this book to the market.

And this undertaking was moved forward by the hard work and assistance of Michael Kogan, graduate of the MHA program at the Texas A&M School of Rural Public Health and a fellow at St. Joseph Medical Center in Houston, Texas, who helped with the research, editing, and interviews so integral to this book.

We thank Don Smithburg, whose experiences leading one of the largest healthcare systems in the United States through the aftermath of Hurricane Katrina inspired us and affected so many. His experiences and personal journey during those dark times are a powerful and valuable lesson for healthcare executives everywhere. We were hopeful for more prominent inclusion of his work; however, we acknowledge his input, which is present throughout this book.

A number of subject matter experts assisted us with this book and co-authored the core content of many chapters, submitted case reviews, or completed interviews of their personal experiences leading their organizations through disasters and catastrophic events. We are grateful for their participation in this work. Short biographies of those who made major contributions to this work follow.

We would also like to acknowledge the following for their contributions to the book and their extraordinary efforts in leading through and responding to crisis situations:

The leadership team at the University of Texas Medical Branch in Galveston, Texas who were so willing to share their experiences and challenges associated with Hurricane Ike.

The entire team at JFK Medical Center in Atlantis Florida for their incredible efforts in responding to the first anthrax event in the United States three weeks after the September 11th attacks. Dr. Larry Bush, CNO Dianne Aleman, vice president of marketing and public relations Madelyn Christopher, and the HCA divisional and corporate staff deserve specific mention.

The Health Science Center and School of Rural Public Health at Texas A&M University for their vision and leadership in developing the next generation of leaders, caregivers, and responders who are so critical to our reaction to and planning for disasters of all types.

Coauthors and Contributors

Those who made major contributions to this work include the following professionals (in alphabetical order):

Leonard Friedman, PhD, MPA, MPH, FACHE

Leonard Friedman is a professor in the department of health services management and leadership at George Washington University. Dr. Friedman has chaired the Health Care Management Division of the Academy of Management and is a member of the governing council at the Institute for Healthcare Improvement's Health Professions Education Collaborative. He has also been board chair of the Association of University Programs in Health Administration. Prior to joining George Washington University, he served as board member at the Oregon Patient Safety Commission and at the Benton County Hospice. He is the recipient of the Regents' Award from the American College of Healthcare Executives.

Dee Grimm, RN, JD

Dee Grimm has over 18 years experience in emergency medicine and 15 years in disaster preparedness/emergency management. She is a registered nurse, and has worked as an emergency management coordinator for several hospitals. She also holds a doctorate of law and provides legal and ethical consulting services. Her consulting firm specializes in disaster preparedness training and emergency management planning consultation. She has served as the project manager for the Nevada Statewide Evacuation, Mass Care, and Sheltering Initiative, conducting evacuation and sheltering plans for the state and its 17 counties. She serves on the initiative's Legal Task Force to make recommendations to the state legislature to amend and improve emergency management statutes. She is also the project manager for the state's Mass Fatality Plan. Grimm teaches at Noble Training Center for FEMA and the Center for Disaster Preparedness. She is a certified instructor in weapons of mass destruction, hospital incident command, haz mat and decon training, and disaster exercise design. She has been a speaker at numerous conferences throughout the country. Grimm is Western Regional director of Pets America, a non-profit organization that promotes pet-friendly sheltering in disasters and disaster preparedness for pets programs.

Melinda Johnson, MPP

Melinda Johnson earned her master's degree in public policy from Regent University and a certification in disaster preparedness from the Milton Hershey School of Medicine at the Pennsylvania State University. She previously worked as director of government affairs for AmerisourceBergen Corporation and has worked for the U.S. House of Representatives and the California State Legislature. As the program coordinator for the Denver Metropolitan Medical Response System, Johnson works closely with the 25 hospitals in the Colorado Front Range Region as well as state and local public health offices in planning and preparing for medical emergencies in the Colorado Front Range. She also serves as a hospital site surveyor for the American College of Emergency Physicians to determine the hospital preparedness levels in select cities across the United States.

Michael Kogan, MHA

Michael Kogan is an administrative fellow at St. Joseph Medical Center in Houston. He has worked in both clinical and administrative settings through-out his undergraduate and graduate careers, gaining experience as an emergency medical technician and as an executive assistant for an orthopaedic surgeon. Kogan received his undergraduate degree in biomedical science from Texas A&M University and his master's in health administration from the Texas A&M School of Rural Public Health.

Jane Kushma, PhD

Jane Kushma has a diverse background in emergency management education and practice. Over the past 15 years she has developed and implemented emergency management degree programs and curricula at the undergraduate and graduate levels at the University of North Texas, University of Tennessee at Chattanooga, and Jacksonville State University in Alabama. She has received research grants in the fields of emergency management and distance learning. Since 1981, Dr. Kushma has also served with the American Red Cross. Her disaster experience includes many large relief operation assignments, catastrophic disaster planning, training and exercise development, and numerous interagency initiatives. She received the FEMA Director's Outstanding Public Service Award in 1994 and a FEMA Special Award in 1993. She is currently an associate professor in the Institute for Emergency Preparedness at Jacksonville State University in Alabama, and serves as the managing editor for the *Journal of Homeland Security and Emergency Management*.

Mitch Saruwatari

Mitch Saruwatari serves as vice president of quality and compliance for LiveProcess, a software company that develops emergency management tools for hospitals and healthcare agencies. He oversees coordination of national healthcare and emergency management standards and interfaces with external organizations. He also works closely with new product development. Prior to this, Saruwatari held response positions within healthcare, public health, and emergency medical services organizations. He has served on several national, state, and local advisory committees, including as co-project manager for the Hospital Incident Command System (HICS). He frequently lectures and instructs on healthcare emergency management issues throughout the nation.

Gregory L. Shaw, DSc, CBCP

Gregory Shaw is an associate professor of engineering management and a co-director of the Institute for Crisis, Disaster, and Risk Management at George Washington University (GWU). He is an adjunct faculty member at Florida Atlantic University and Massachusetts Maritime Academy, where he teaches graduate level courses in homeland security, crisis and emergency management, and risk management. Shaw previously served as an officer in the U.S. Coast Guard, retiring as a captain in October 1996. While on active duty, he commanded four cutters and the Coast Guard's largest shore unit, served as director of training and education, and served as a senior analyst for a congressionally chartered commission. He earned a doctorate of science in engineering management at George Washington University and masters' degrees in physics at Wesleyan University, education and human development at GWU, and business administration at Webster University. He is a certified business continuity professional (CBCP) through Disaster Recovery Institute International.

Donald Smithburg

Donald Smithburg served as CEO of the nine-hospital LSU-Charity Hospital System during Hurricanes Katrina and Rita. Those catastrophes devastated the system's flagship in New Orleans known as Big Charity, where most of the region's low income citizens received their care. Massive complex evacuations, loss of 90 percent of its workforce, development of major interim facilities, and long-term recovery of the healthcare infrastructure amidst extraordinary community disaster consumed Smithburg's leadership responsibilities. Prior to the Charity Hospital System, Smithburg was a leader of the public hospital system of Kansas City, MO and served as chief administrative officer for the University of Missouri-Kansas City School of Medicine. He also was president/CEO of the University of Texas at Southwestern Hospitals in Dallas. He currently is executive associate dean at Florida International University College of Medicine in Miami, FL and also is a consultant to healthcare organizations.

G. Edward Tucker, Jr., CPA, CMC

Ed Tucker has over 40 years' experience in healthcare financial management, including stints in senior management of hospitals and Blue Cross & Blue Shield plans. Tucker is a CPA and certified management consultant. He served on the American Institute of CPAs' Health Care Committee and is an active member of the Healthcare Financial Management Association. Tucker was chief financial manager of Forrest General Hospital, a 512-bed level II trauma center in Hattiesburg, MS, when Hurricane Katrina struck. Tucker dealt with Katrina's physical and fiscal aftermath, including extensive damage to his own home.

Brent H. Woodworth

Brent Woodworth is a well known leader in global risk and crisis management. In December 2007 he retired from IBM after 32 years of service, which included the development and management of all worldwide crisis response team operations. Woodworth founded and managed the Crisis Response Team—a team of international specialists focused on helping governments and businesses prepare for, respond to, and recover from catastrophic events. He also created the SAHANA international emergency management system, an open-source system currently running in 17 countries. Woodworth also has served on the Congressional subcommittee for the development of the national pre-disaster mitigation plan, the board of the U.S. Multihazard Mitigation Council, and the board of the National Institute of Building Sciences. He is currently CEO of the LA Preparedness Foundation.

Interviewees

Those who contributed by submitting responses to questions concerning their experiences leading their organizations through significant events include the following:

David Callendar, MD, MBA, FACS

David Callendar became president of the University of Texas Medical Branch in Galveston on September 1, 2007. Dr. Callender served as the associate vice chancellor and CEO for the UCLA Hospital System from mid 2004 to 2007. A 1984 graduate of Baylor College of Medicine, he completed his residency training in general surgery and otolaryngology at his alma mater in 1990. He has authored a number of scientific and educational publications. Dr. Callender received an MBA from the University of Houston in 1995.

Timothy L. Charles

Timothy L. Charles is the chief executive officer of Mercy Medical Center in Cedar Rapids, Iowa, a position he has held since 2003. He previously served as executive vice president at Mercy, and was CEO of Denton Community Hospital in Denton, IA from 1997 to 2003.

Beth Ingram

Beth Ingram is vice president of the Arkansas Hospital Association in Little Rock, where she has been employed since 1978. In addition to editing the AHA's quarterly publications *Arkansas Hospitals* and *The Arkansas Trustee*, and managing the association's annual meeting and summer conference, her responsibilities include managing the association's education program, governance, and emergency preparedness issues. She holds a bachelor of arts degree from the University of Arkansas at Little Rock. Ingram is a member of the American College of Healthcare Executives and the Arkansas Society of Association Executives, board member of the Arkansas Health Executives forum, and past-president of the Arkansas Rural Health Forum and Executive Women International. She also is a board member of the Twentieth Century Club in Little Rock, a philanthropic organization

Michael J. Megna, FACHE

Michael J. Megna is associate vice president of business operations and facilities and institutional emergency preparedness officer at the University of Texas Medical Branch at Galveston. Megna has over 28 years of service with the university, including time as executive director for UTMB hospitals and administrator of the Orthopaedics and Rehabilitation Department. He is responsible for operations and planning for UTMB facilities and campus services, maintaining the University Master Facilities Plan, and for all aspects of institutional facility planning for internal customers. As institutional emergency preparedness officer he is responsible for developing and maintaining institutional disaster response plans and evacuation plans, and assuring compliance with legal and external accreditation requirements related to emergency preparedness.

Kirk Reamey, FACHE

Herbert K. Reamey III (Kirk) has been the CEO of Ozark Health in Clinton, AR since May 2005. Prior to his current position, Reamey was the CEO of Magnolia City Hospital, Magnolia, AR for over seven years. Reamey is an at-large delegate to the Arkansas Hospital Association Board of Directors, and represented rural hospitals on the American Hospital Association's Region 7 Policy Board from 2005 to 2008. Kirk is a past president of the Arkansas Hospital Administrators Forum.

Angela Richmond, MBA, FACHE

Angela Richmond is president and CEO of the Community Medical Center of Izard County. Previously, she simultaneously ran her current hospital and Fulton County Hospital. In this joint position, Richmond opened a new facility, salvaged a bottom line, and reported to two hospital boards. Richmond began her healthcare career as director of finance for Ozarks Medical Center in West Plains, MO.

Windsor Westbrook Sherrill, PhD

Windsor Westbrook Sherrill is an associate professor in public health sciences at Clemson University. She has worked in health administration at the Medical College of Georgia Hospital, and served as a consultant in the assessment and evaluation of health delivery systems for the Picker Institute for Patient Centered Care, the Hawaii Health Services System, and Health Decisions, Inc. of New Jersey. She obtained a doctorate in health policy from the Florence Heller School of Brandeis University. She has graduate degrees in health services administration and business administration from the University of Alabama at Birmingham.

Randall Wright, FACHE

Randall Wright has served in various positions at Texas Children's Hospital since 2000; he became chief operating officer in 2005. Prior to joining Texas Children's Hospital, Wright held executive roles at the Methodist Hospital in Houston for 20 years. Wright has a master's degree in business administration and is a certified public accountant. He has served as chairman of the board of LifeGift, the organ procurement organization that supports many of the organ transplant programs in Texas.

About the Authors

K. Joanne McGlown, Ph.D, MHHA, RN, FACHE

Dr. McGlown is the global business development director for Sigma Theta Tau International, the Honor Society of Nursing, in Indianapolis, IN. Prior to 2010, she spent 17 years as chief executive officer of McGlown-Self Consulting in Montevallo, Alabama; and as a subject matter expert and consultant to healthcare organizations and facilities in mitigation of, preparedness for, response to, and recovery from disasters and catastrophic events. She continues as a disaster and healthcare consultant with Argonne National Laboratory, and adjunct professor at the University of Alabama at Birmingham. For six years, she was a subject matter expert and course faculty at the Department of Homeland Security/FEMA's Noble Training Facility. Dr. McGlown has more than 35 years experience in pre-hospital emergency medical services (EMS), nursing, and healthcare administration, and also has broad teaching experience in the areas of EMS, emergency and disaster management, and healthcare delivery in emergency and disaster environments. Her work has involved clinical and administrative management and consulting in the public, private, and government sectors. Dr. McGlown holds degrees in emergency medical services and fire science administration, a bachelor's degree in sociology/psychology, and a master of science degree in hospital and health administration. Her doctorate is in administration of health services, with a major in strategic management. She has served on many national and international emergency management committees and participates in a number of task forces and think-tank meetings in these topic areas. Dr. McGlown is board chairman of the Emergency Information Infrastructure Partnership (EIIP), a past board member and officer of the World Association of Disaster and Emergency Medicine (WADEM), and a frequent national and international speaker and lecturer on a variety of topics, including hospital preparedness for disasters and terrorism. She is editor of *Terrorism and Disaster Management: Preparing Healthcare Leaders for the New Reality* (Health Administration Press, 2004).

Phillip Robinson, MHA, FACHE

A native Houstonian and a graduate of Texas A&M University, Phil Robinson received his masters in health administration from Washington University in St. Louis Missouri. He has spent over 30 years in leadership roles in both for-profit and not-for-profit hospitals, including The Methodist Hospital in Houston, the Ochsner Foundation Hospital in New Orleans, HCA, and most recently St. Joseph Medical Center in Houston. He was honored in 2007 as the distinguished alumnus from Washington University's Health Administration Program for his dedication to the university and accomplishments to the field. He was also selected as a *Modern Healthcare* "Up and Comer" in 1992. He has served as the American College of Healthcare Executives (ACHE) regent for East Florida, and lectured frequently at ACHE events. He has served as adjunct faculty at the Washington University Health Administration Program, Florida Atlantic University, and Texas A&M University. He was a founding member of the board of the LifeGift Organ Donation Center and a former chairman of its board.

Robinson's extensive experience leading healthcare organizations during crisis situations includes several hurricanes. He also was CEO of JFK Medical Center in Atlantis, Florida, which admitted the first victim of the anthrax attack three weeks after September 11, 2001. His interest in the impact of disasters began when he visited Russia and the Ukraine in the early 1990s. There he visited hospitals where the victims of the Chernobyl accident were being treated. He subsequently served on the board of the International Consortium on the Long Term Effects of Exposure to Low-Dose Radiation.

Notes

Notes

Notes

Notes